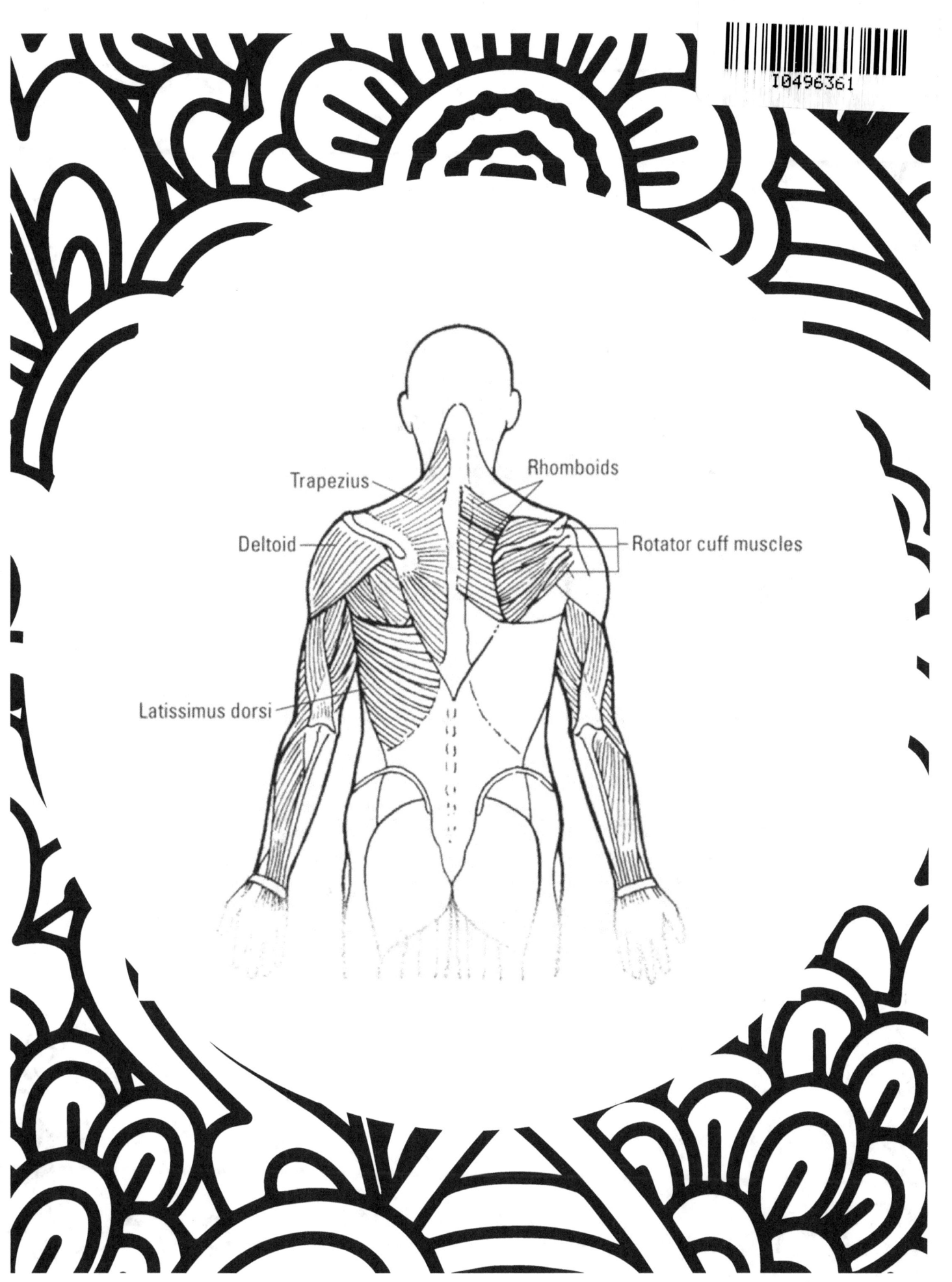

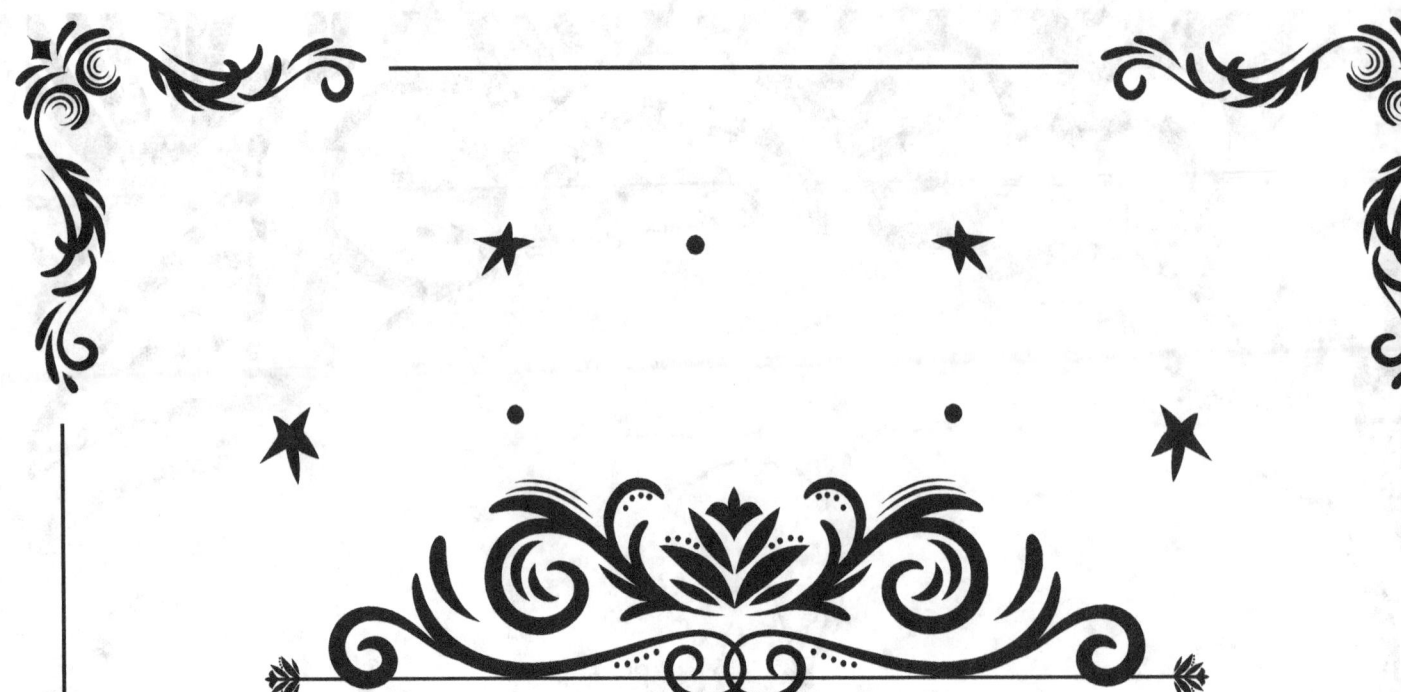

This Book Belongs To

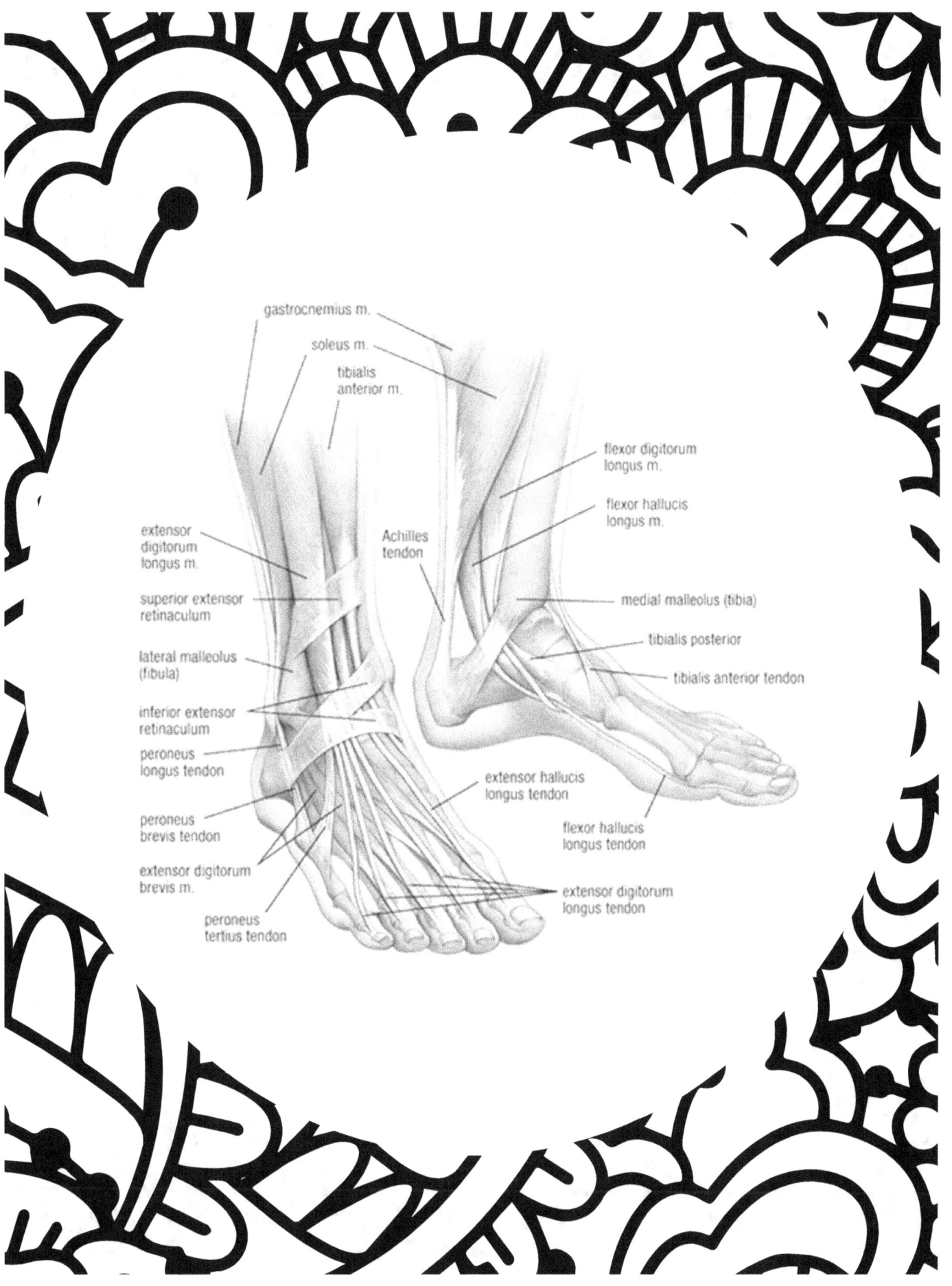

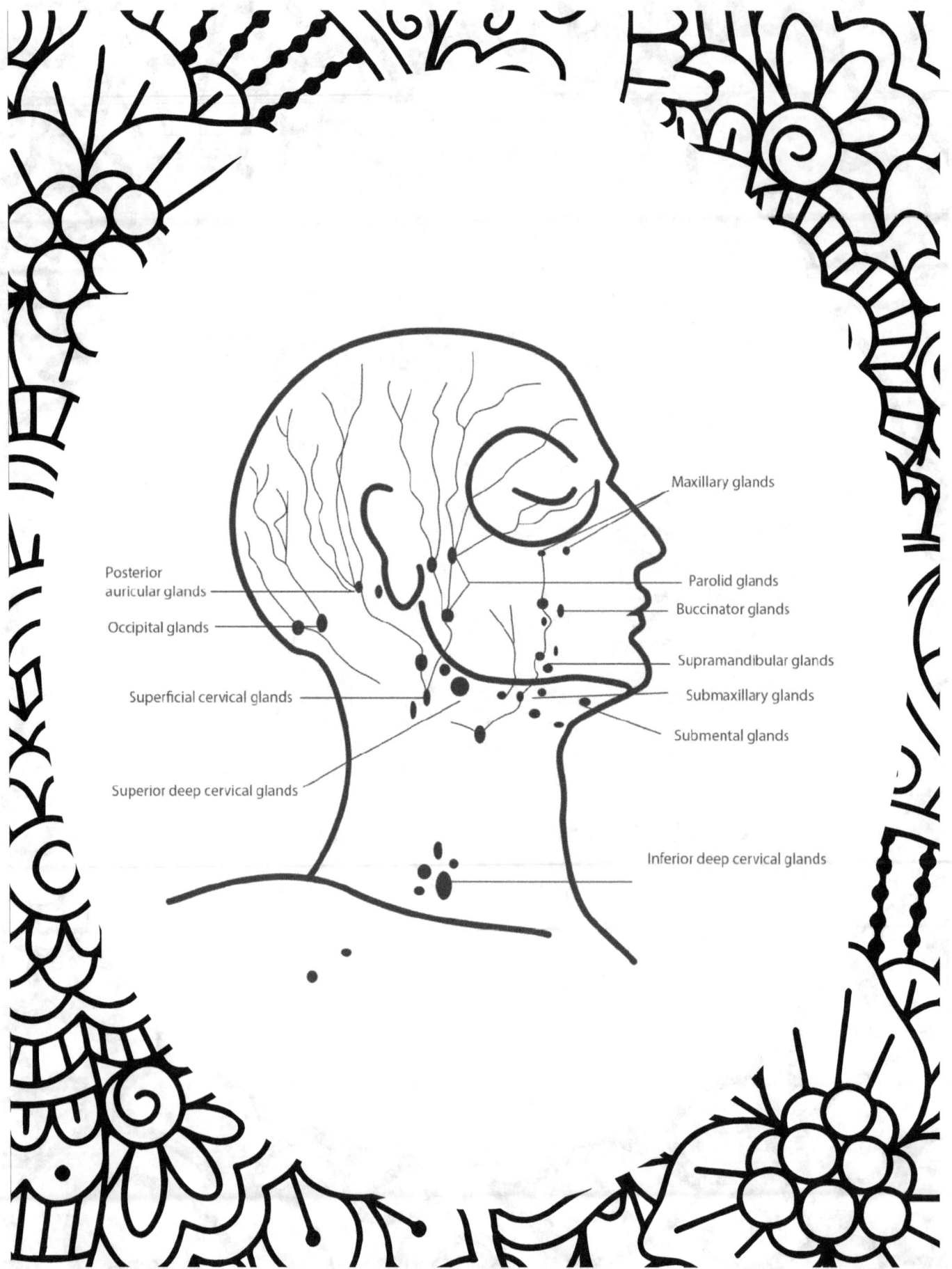

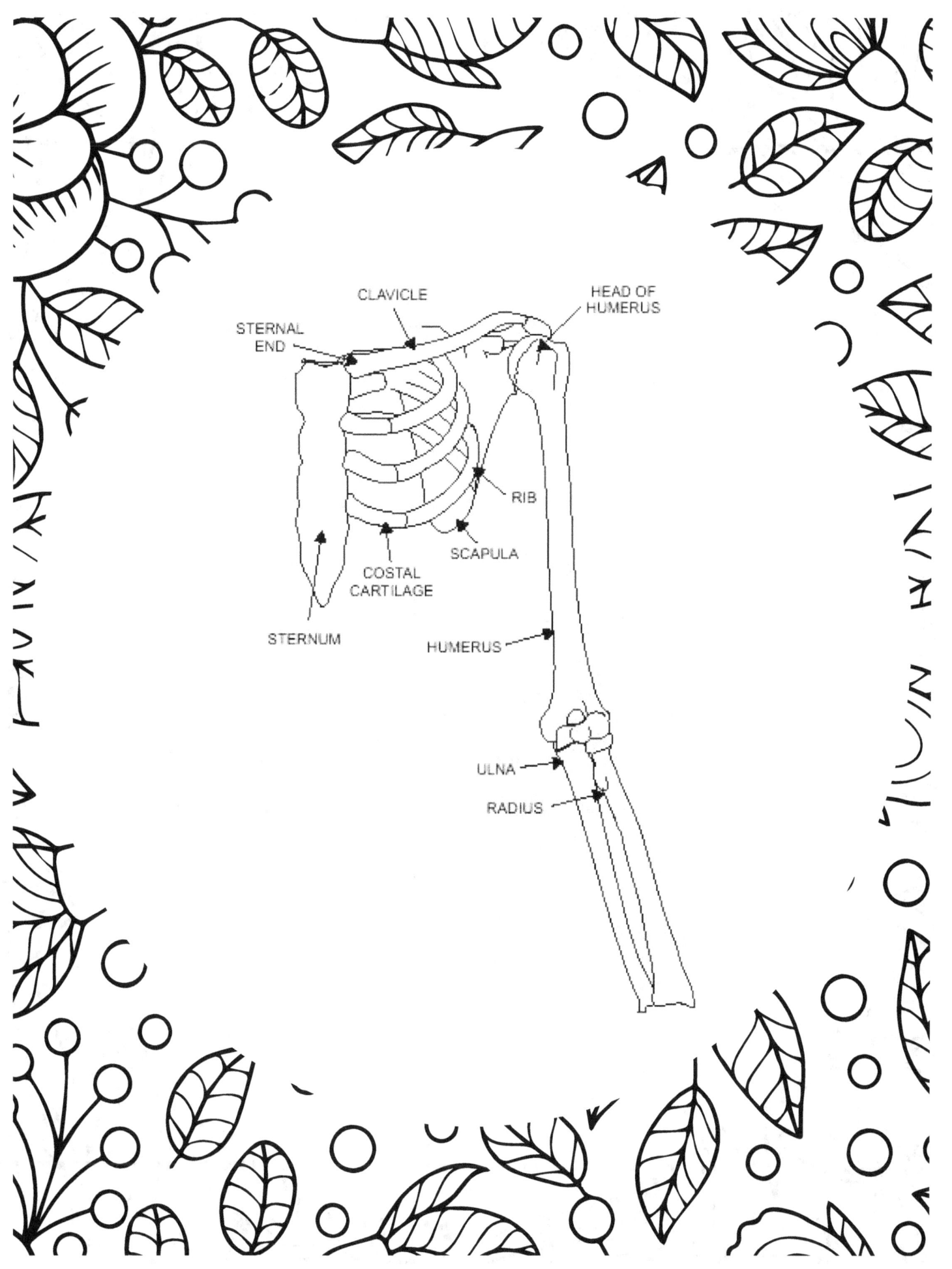

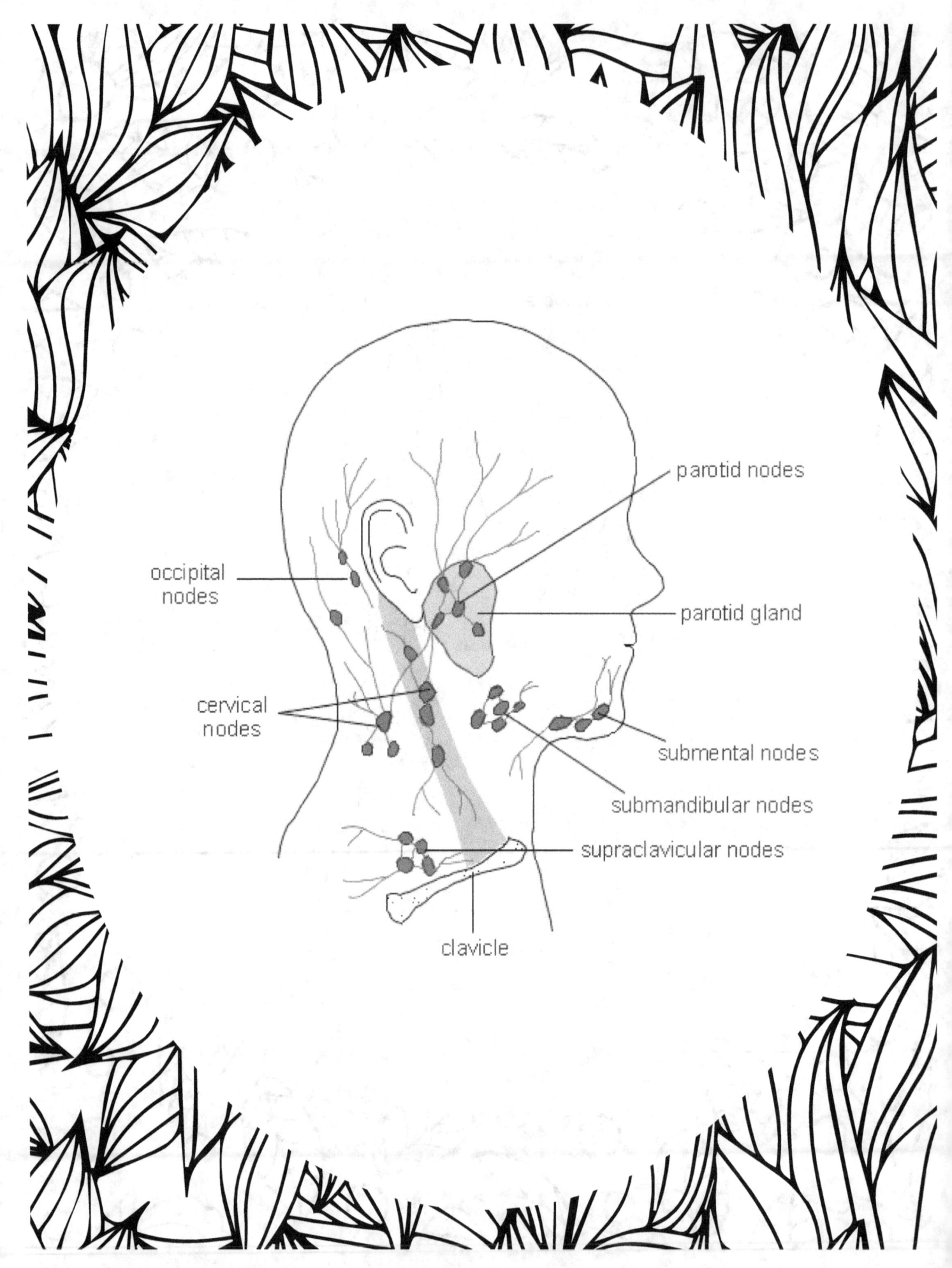

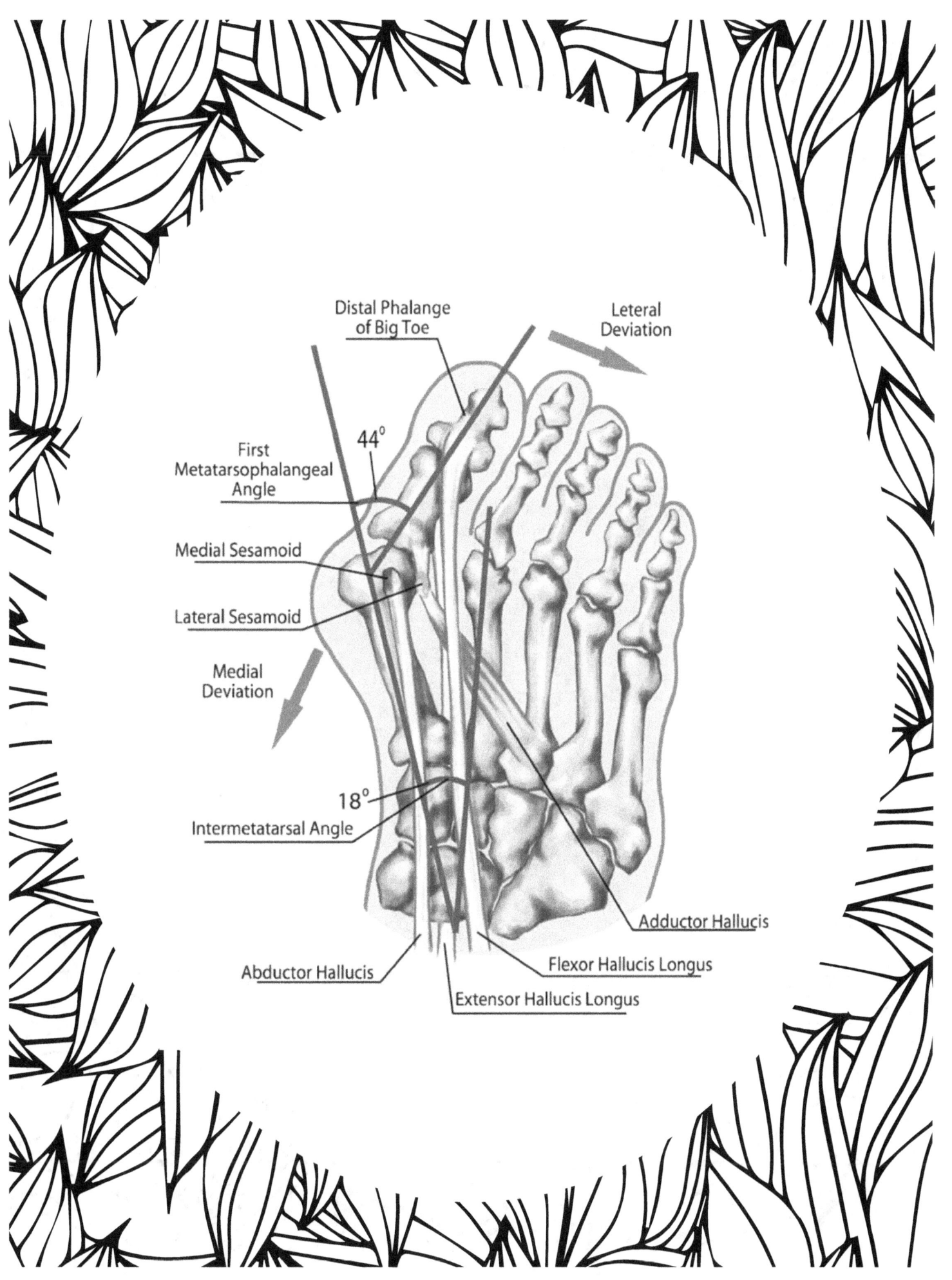

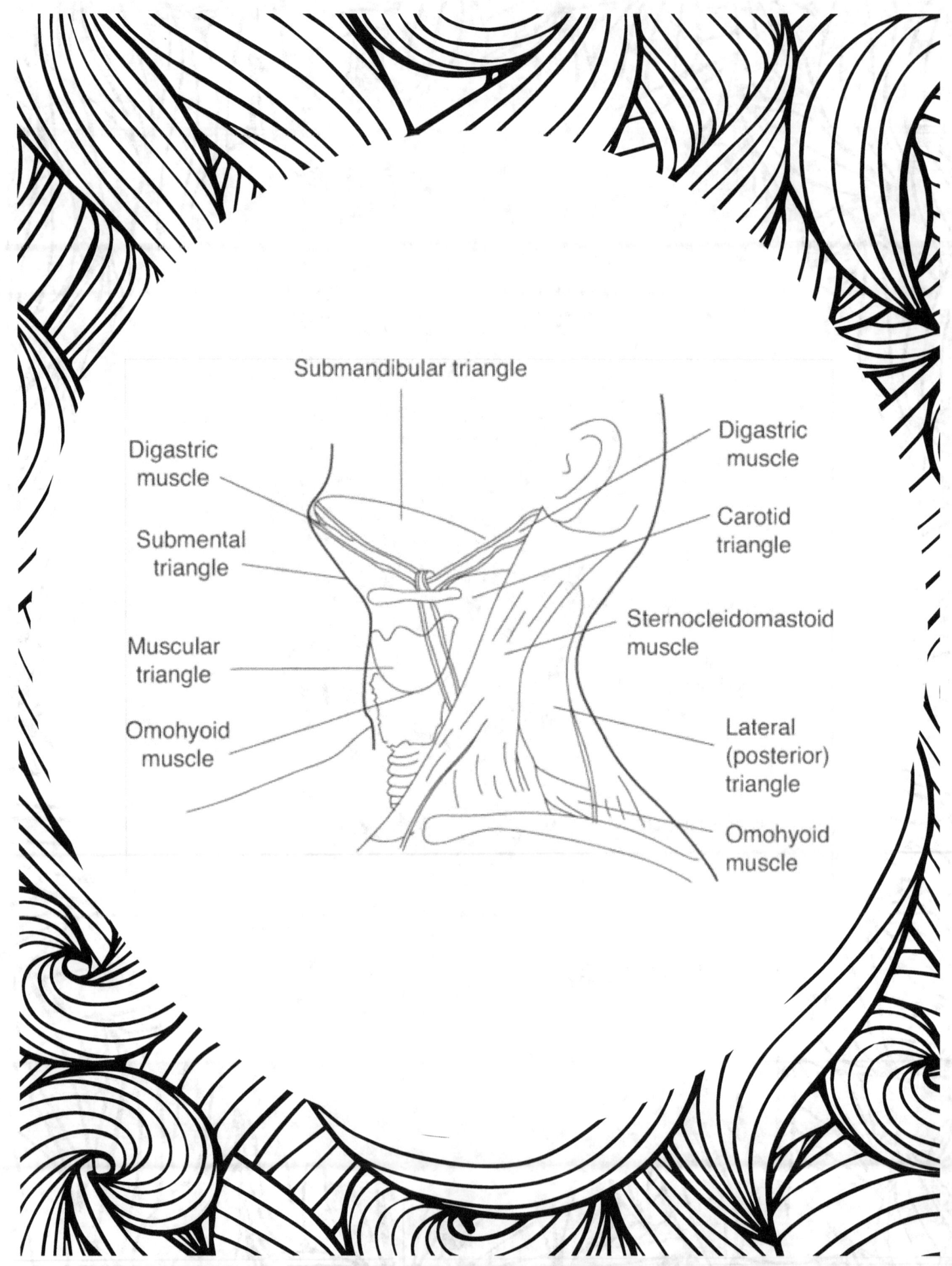

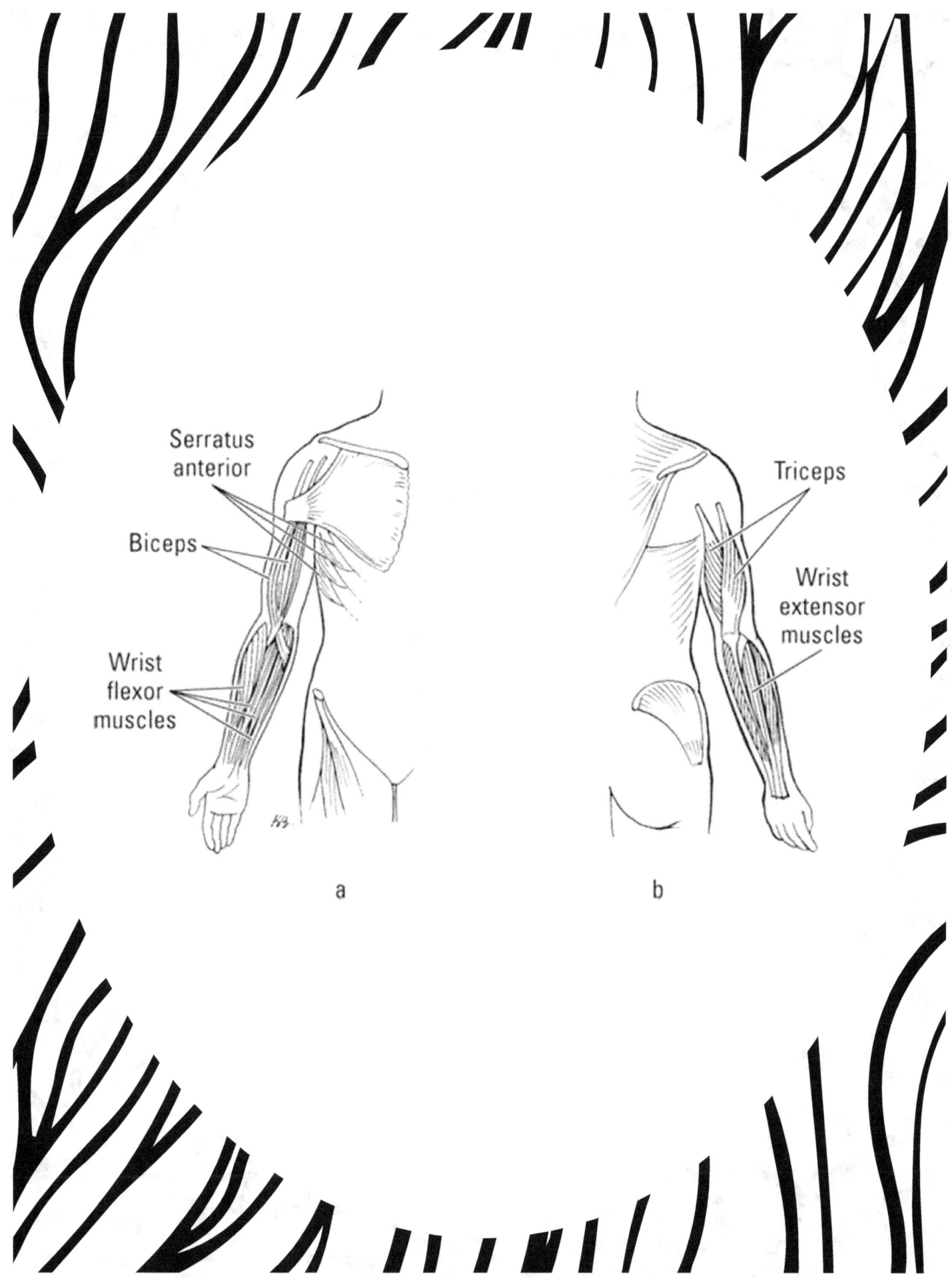

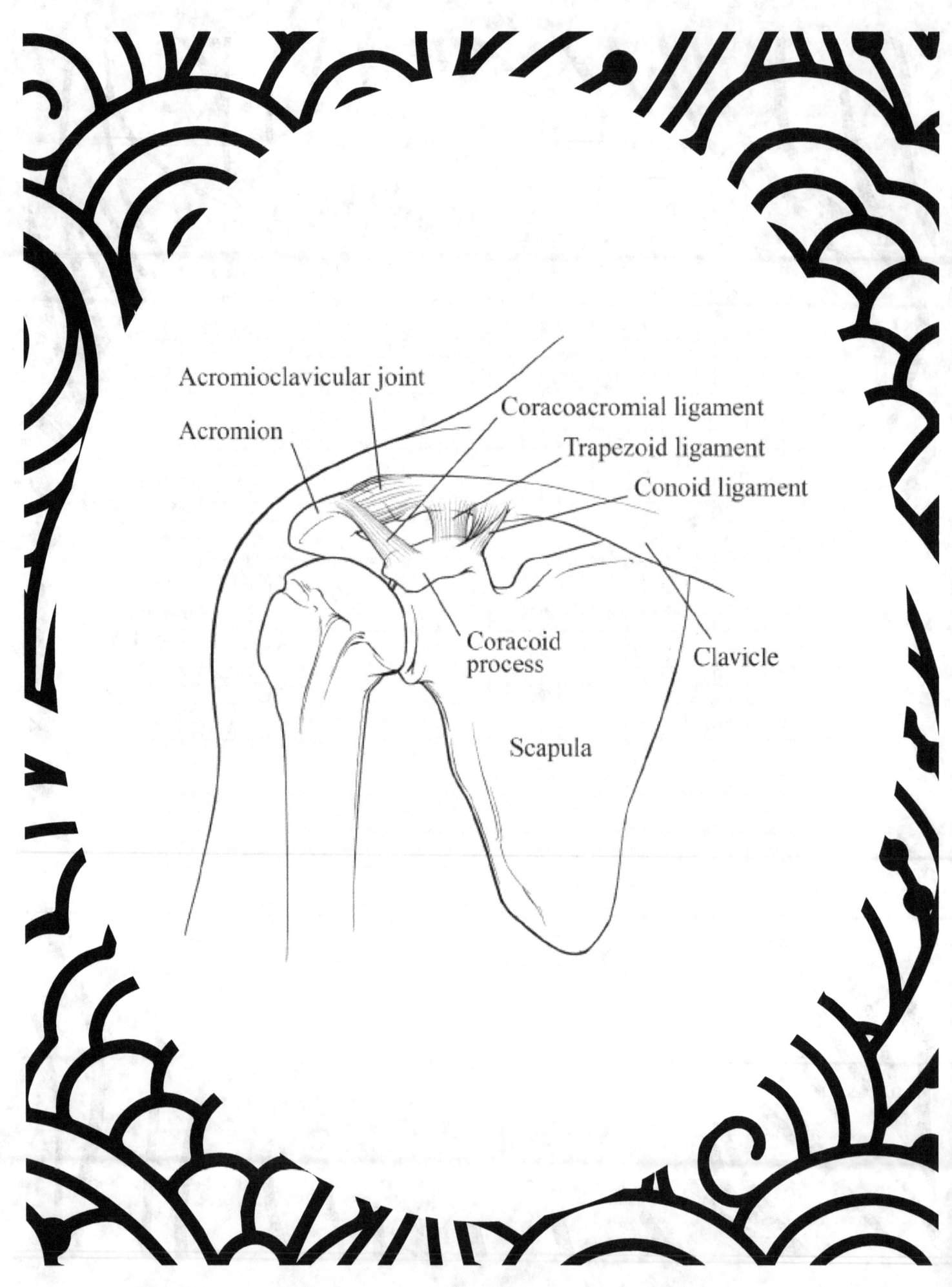

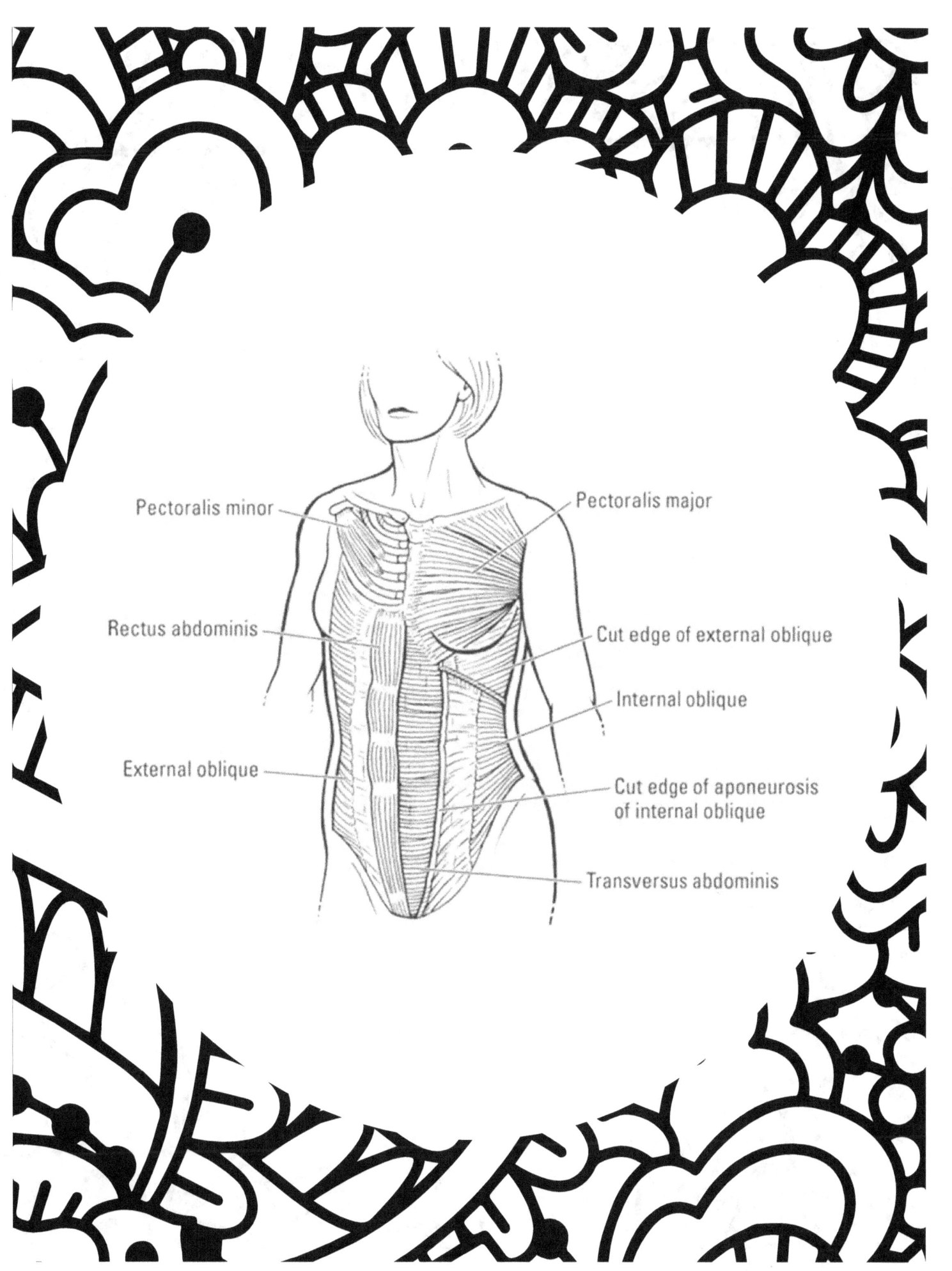

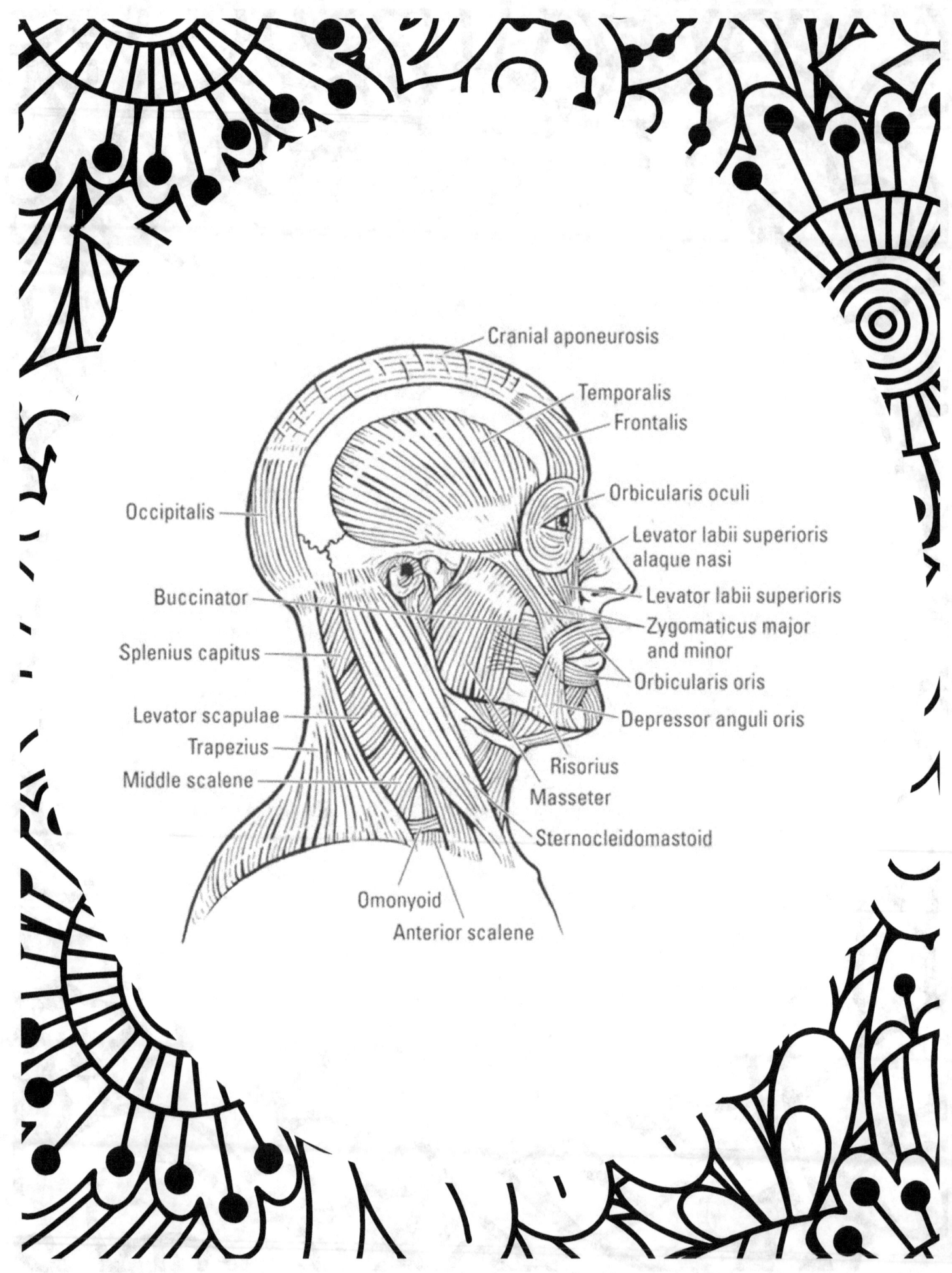

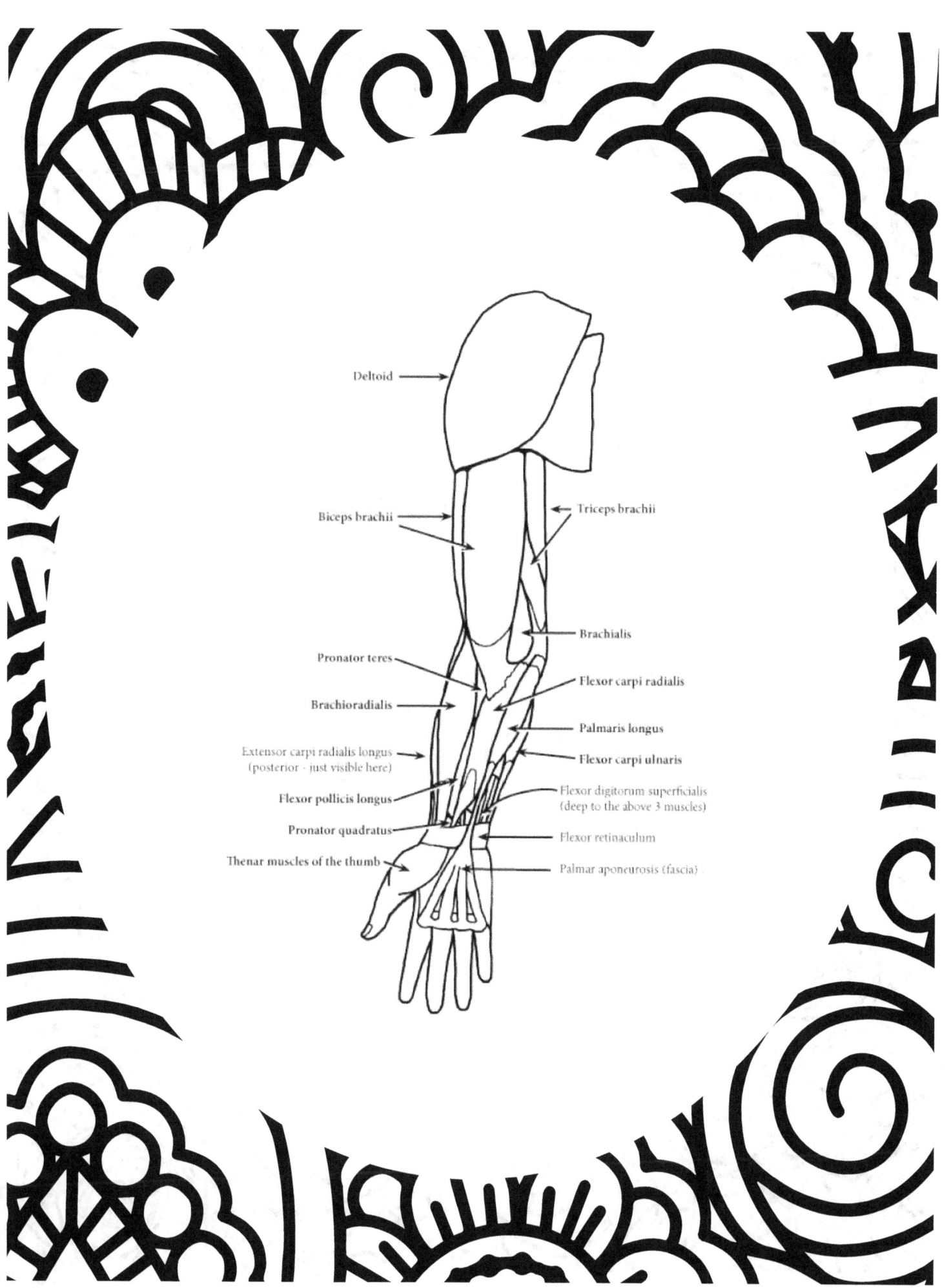

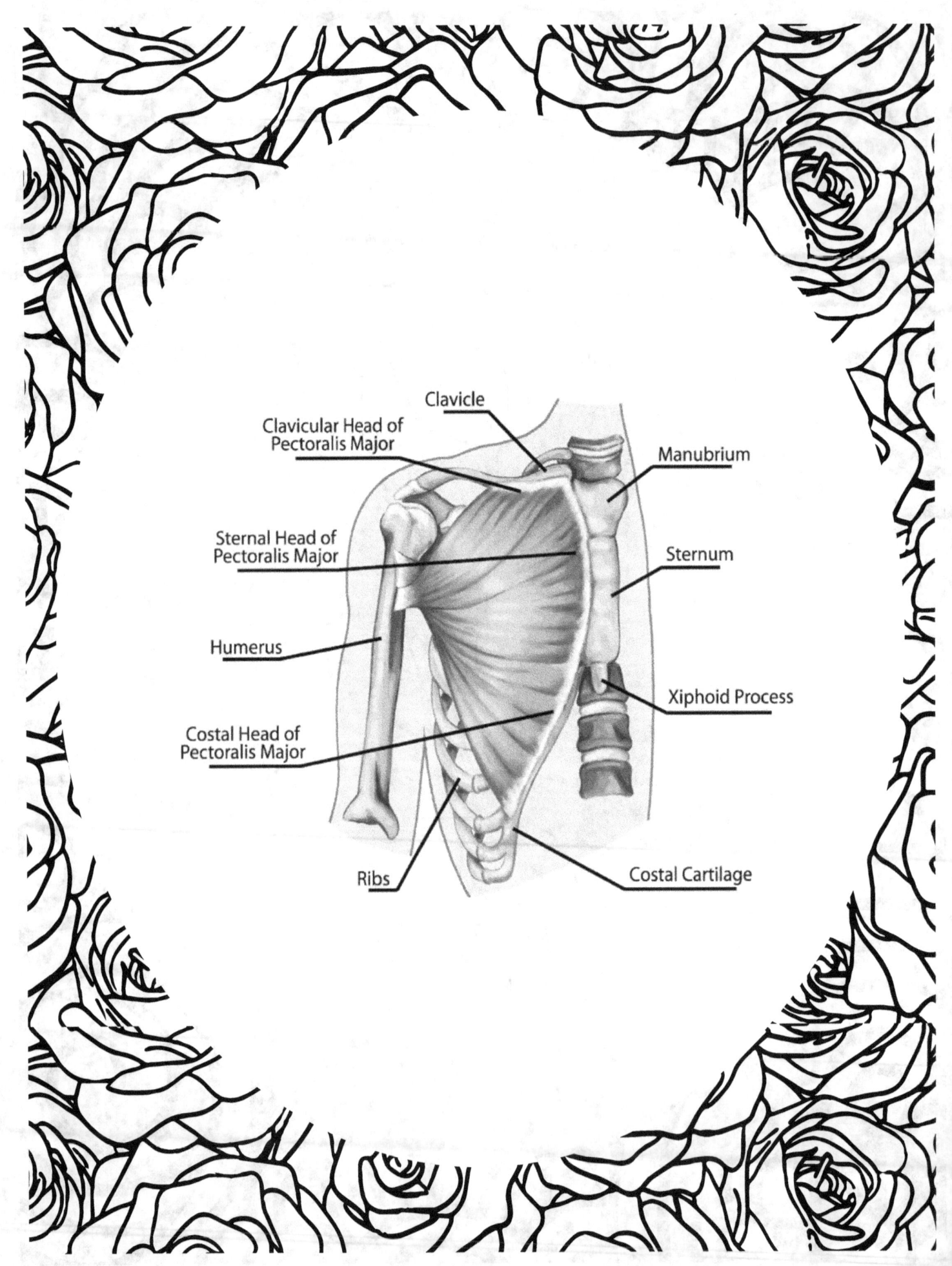

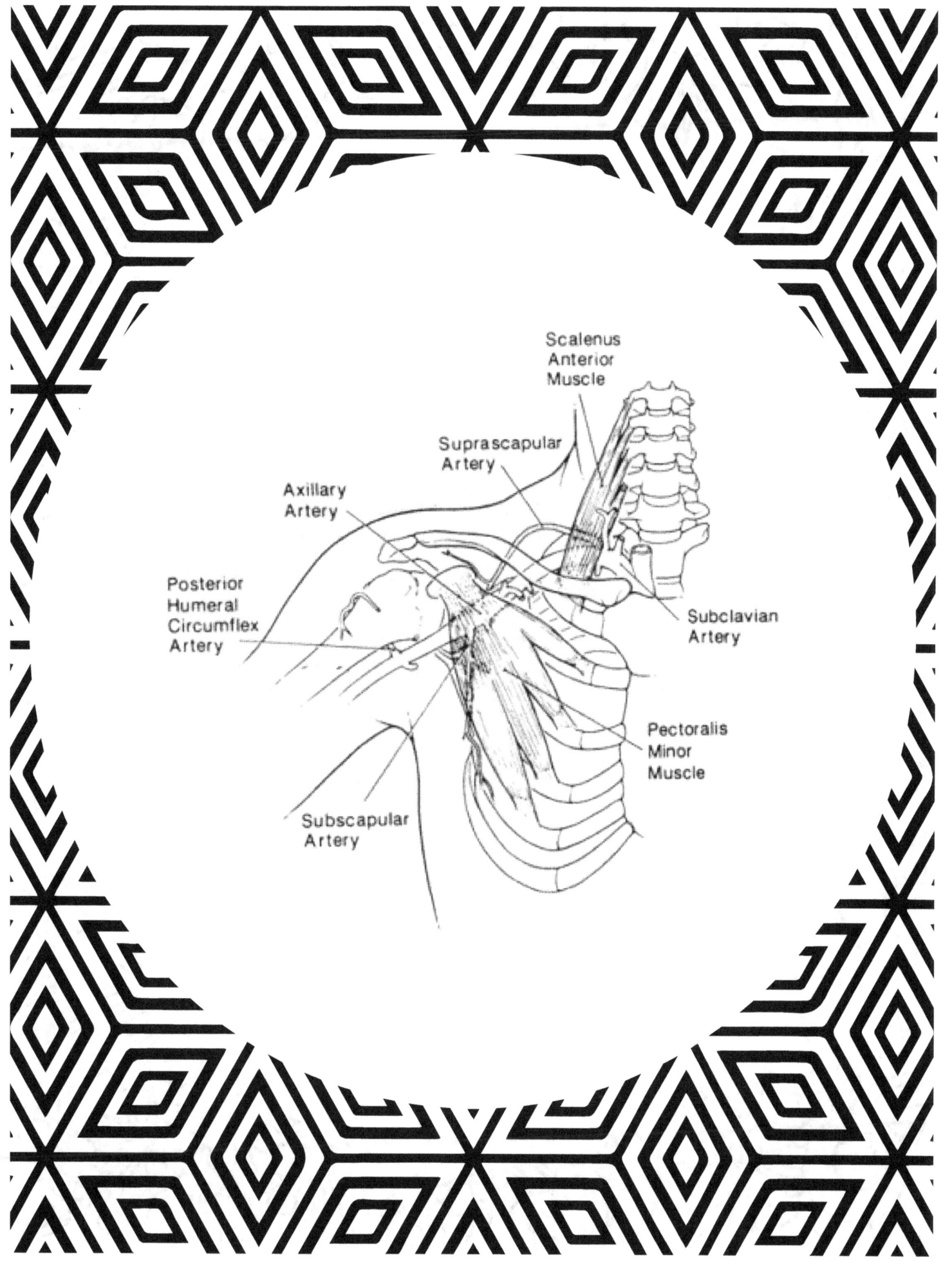

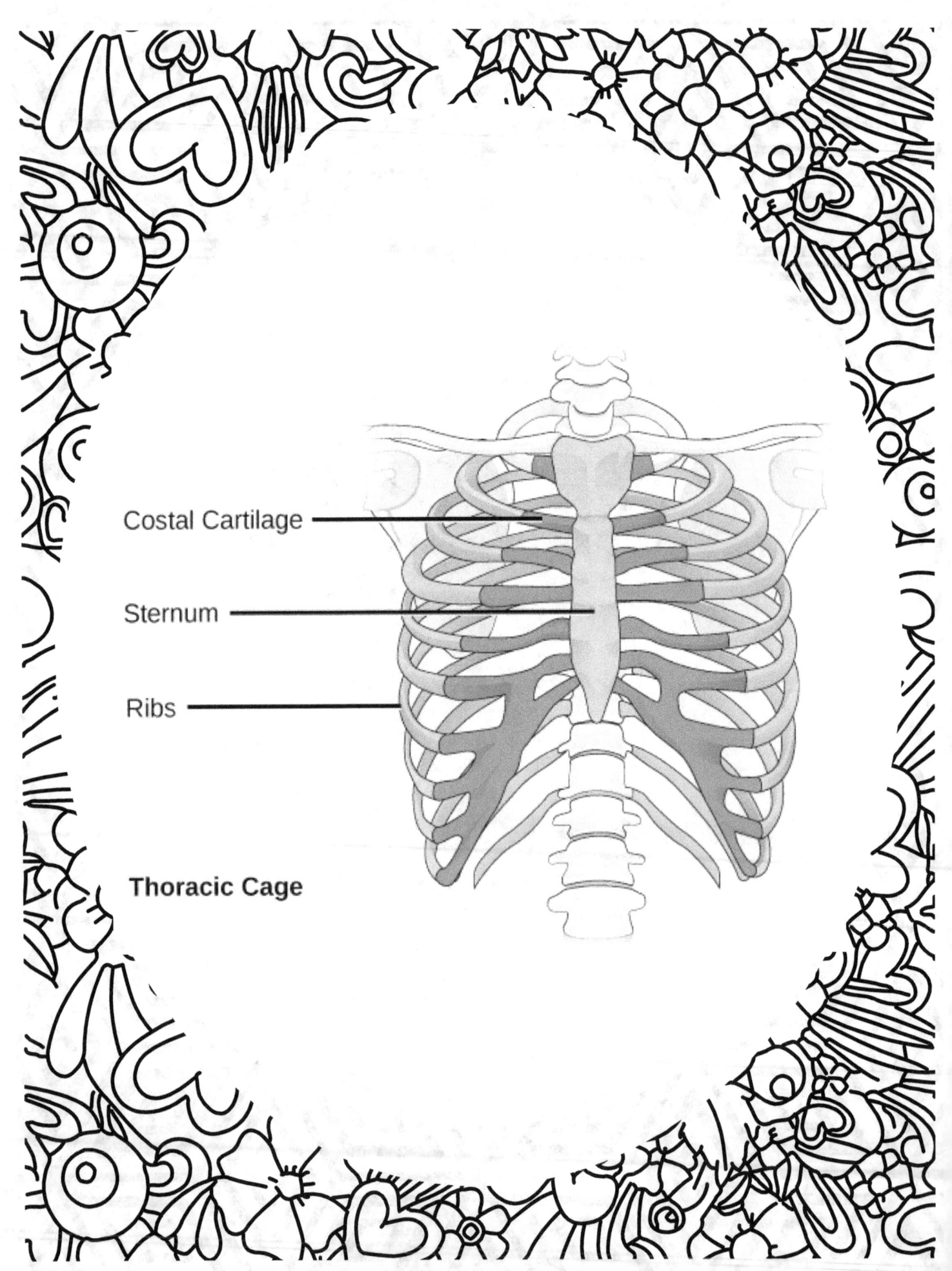

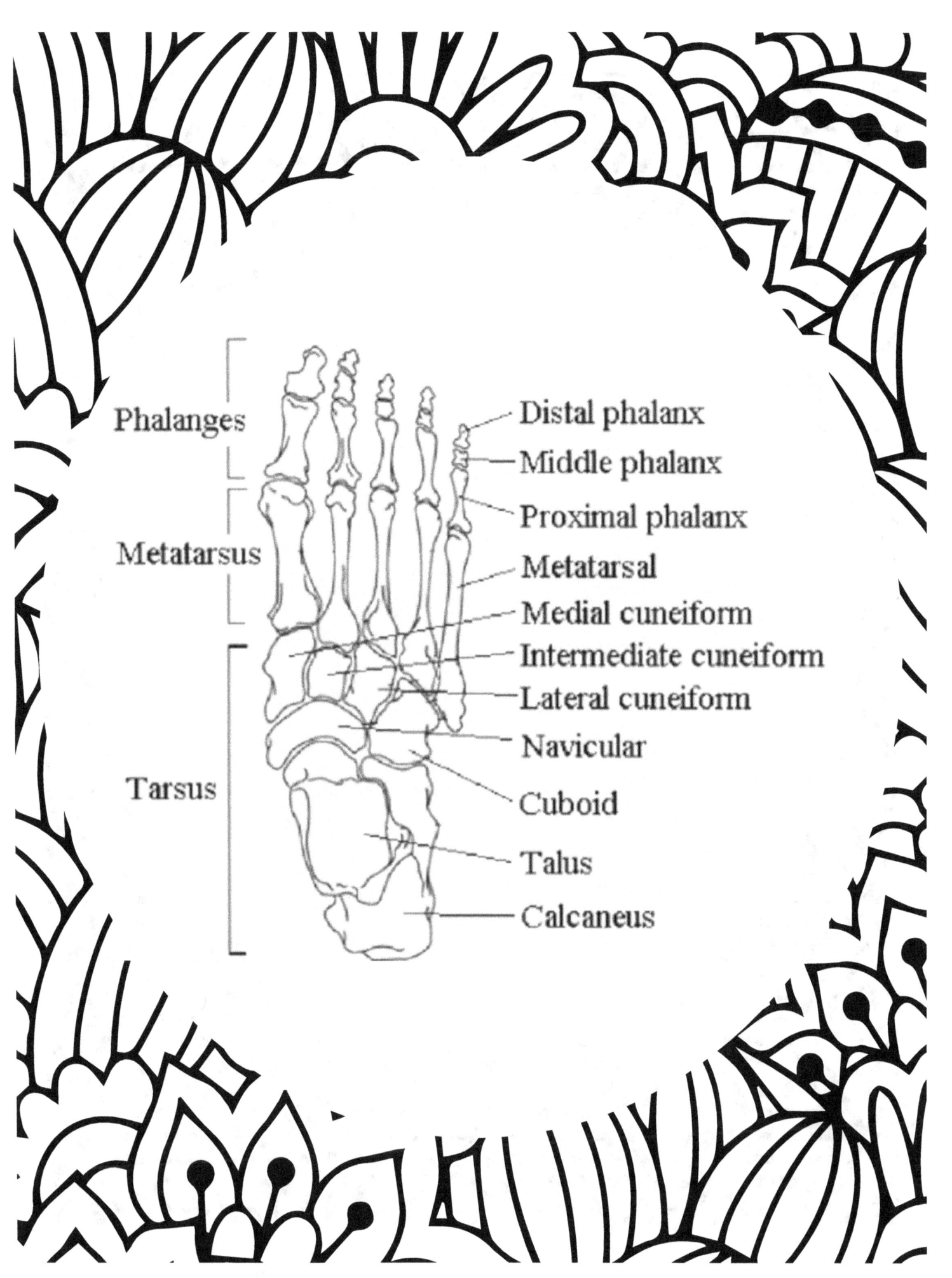

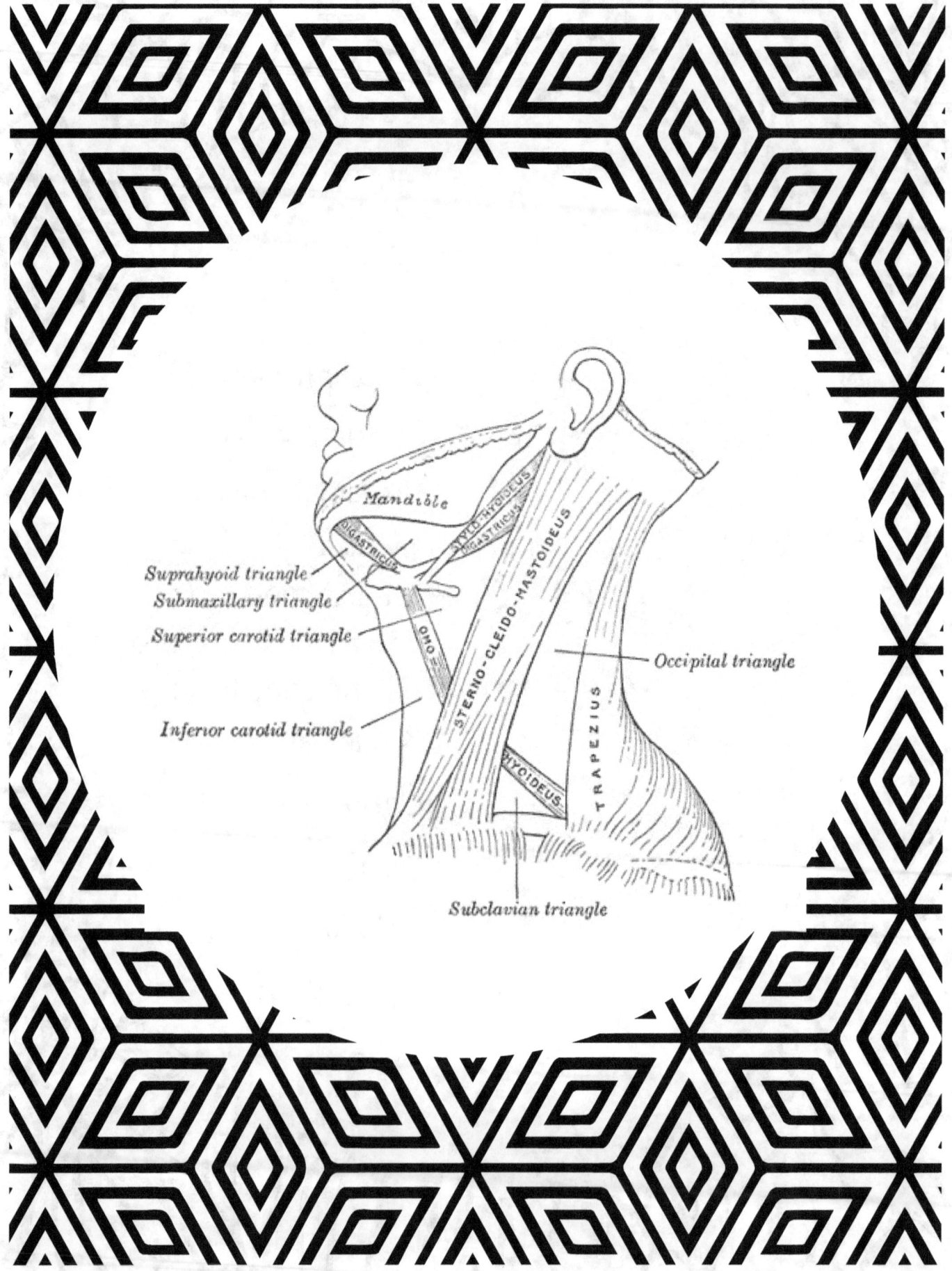

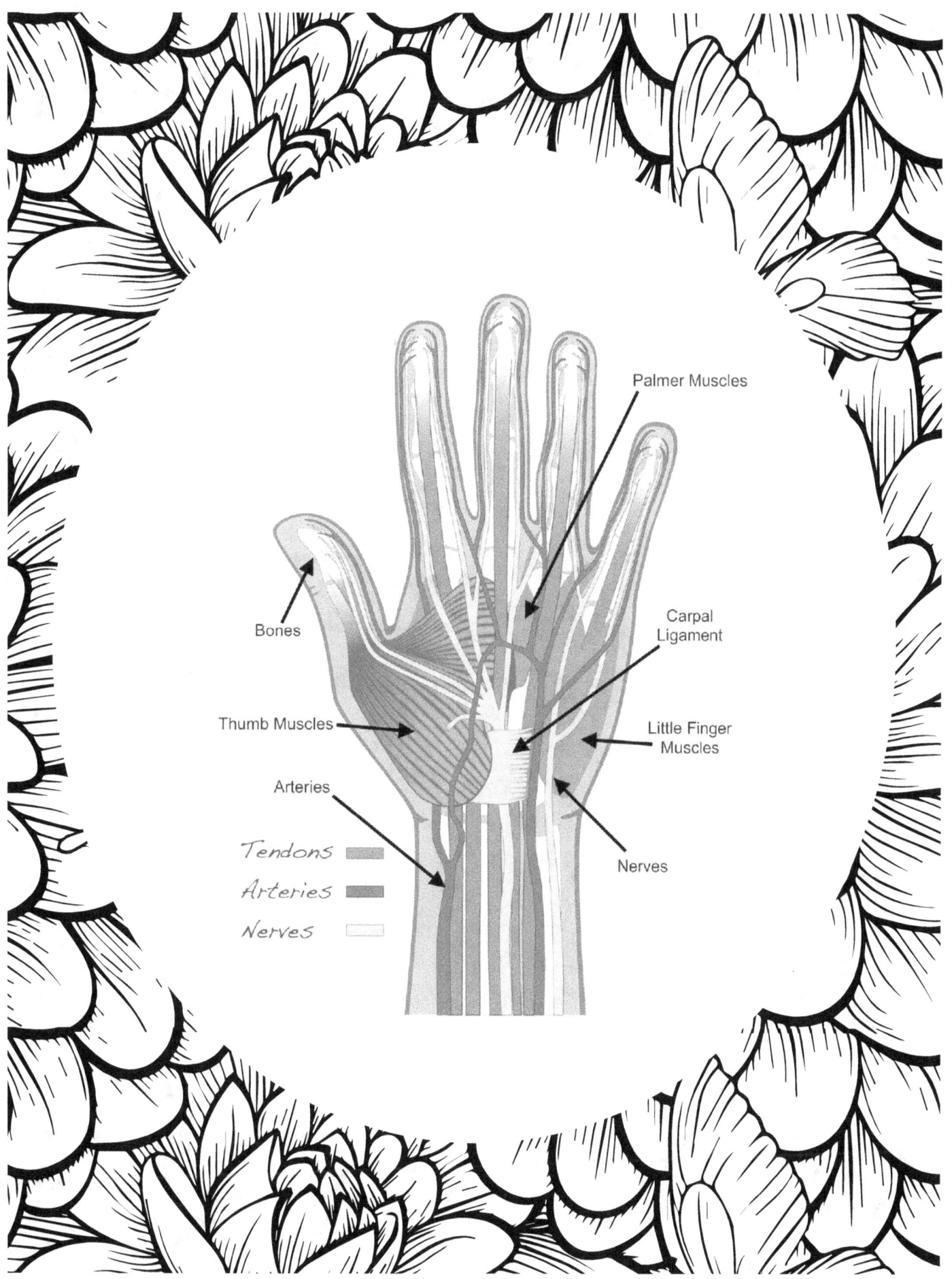

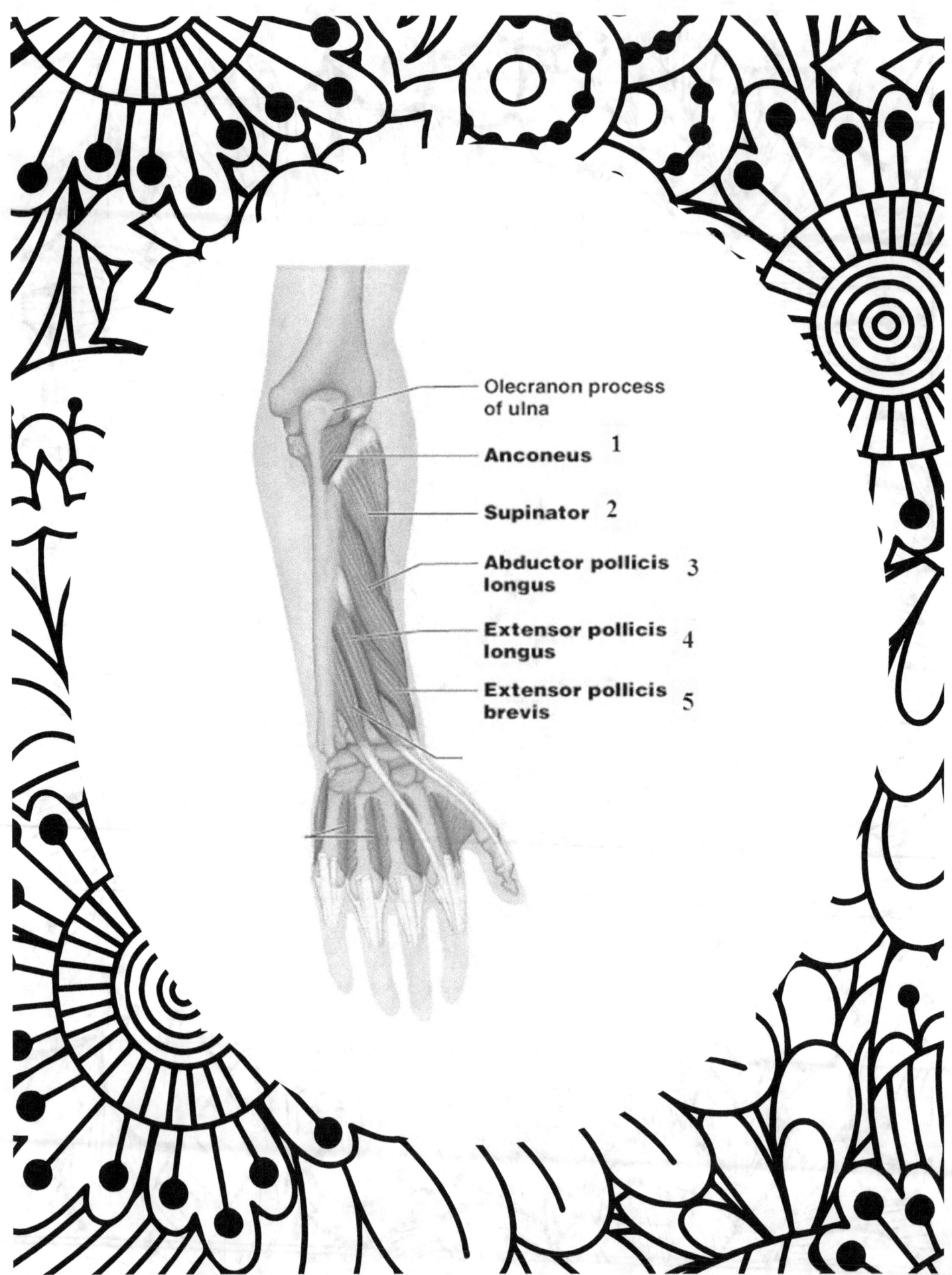

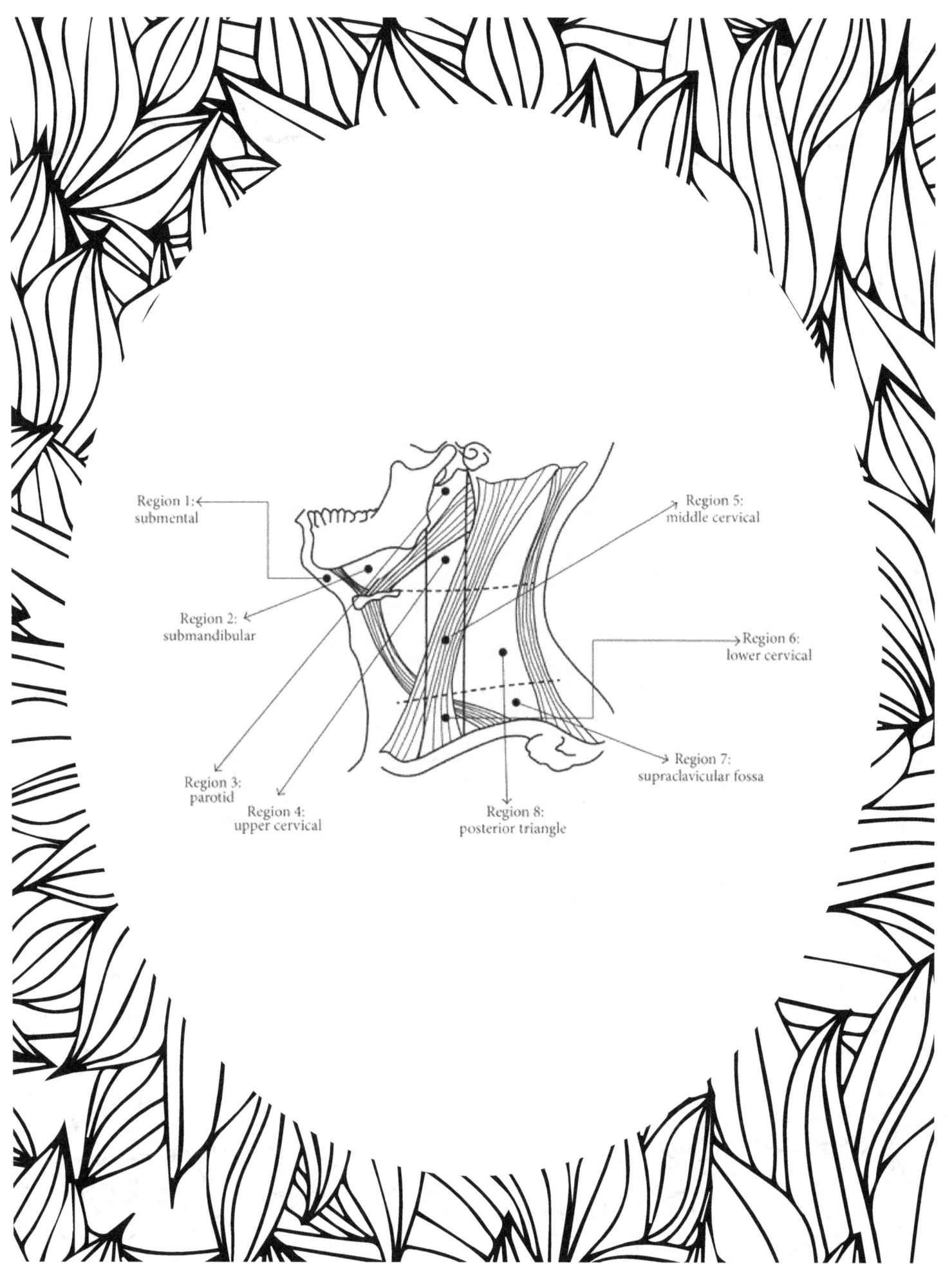

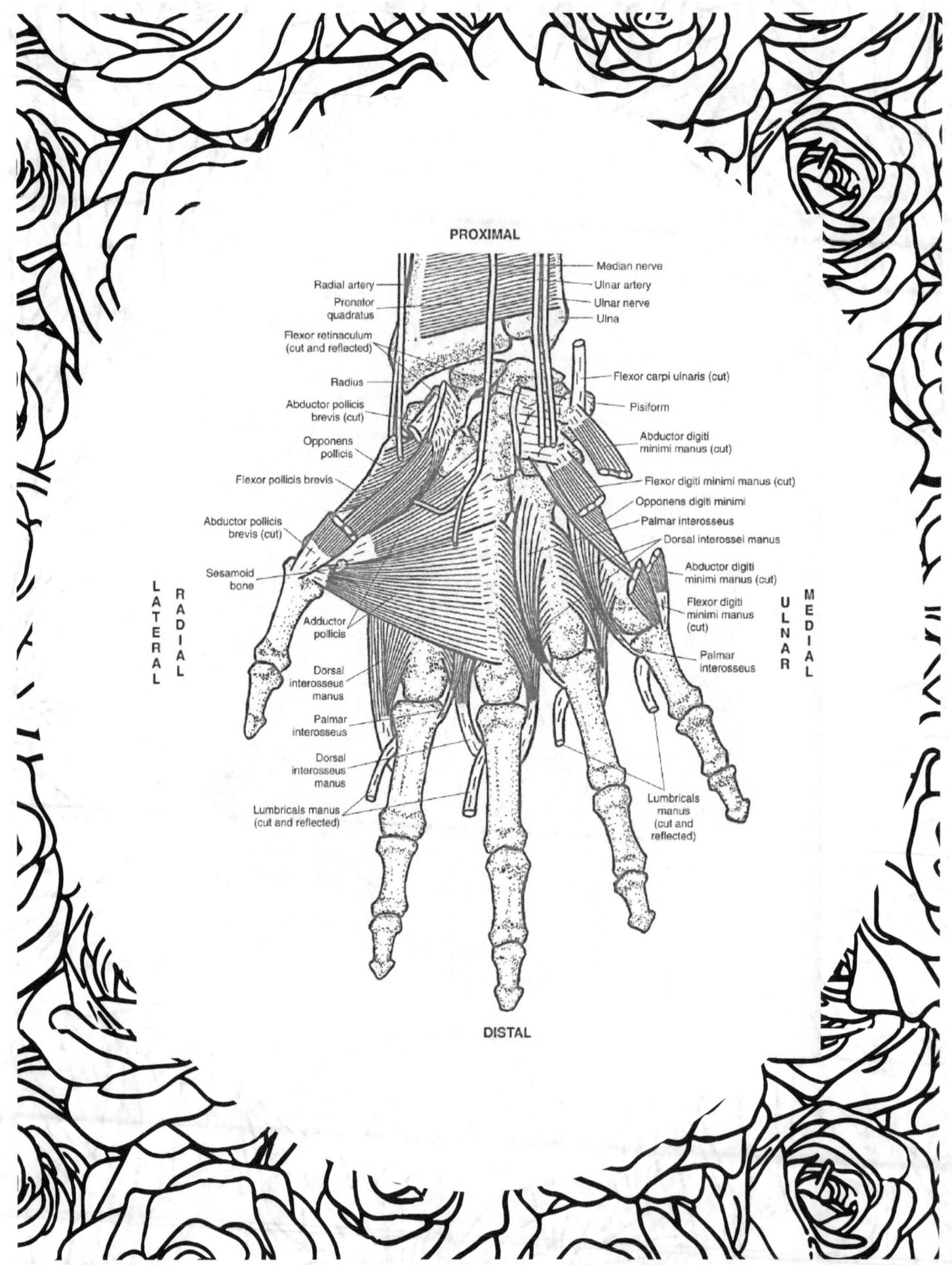

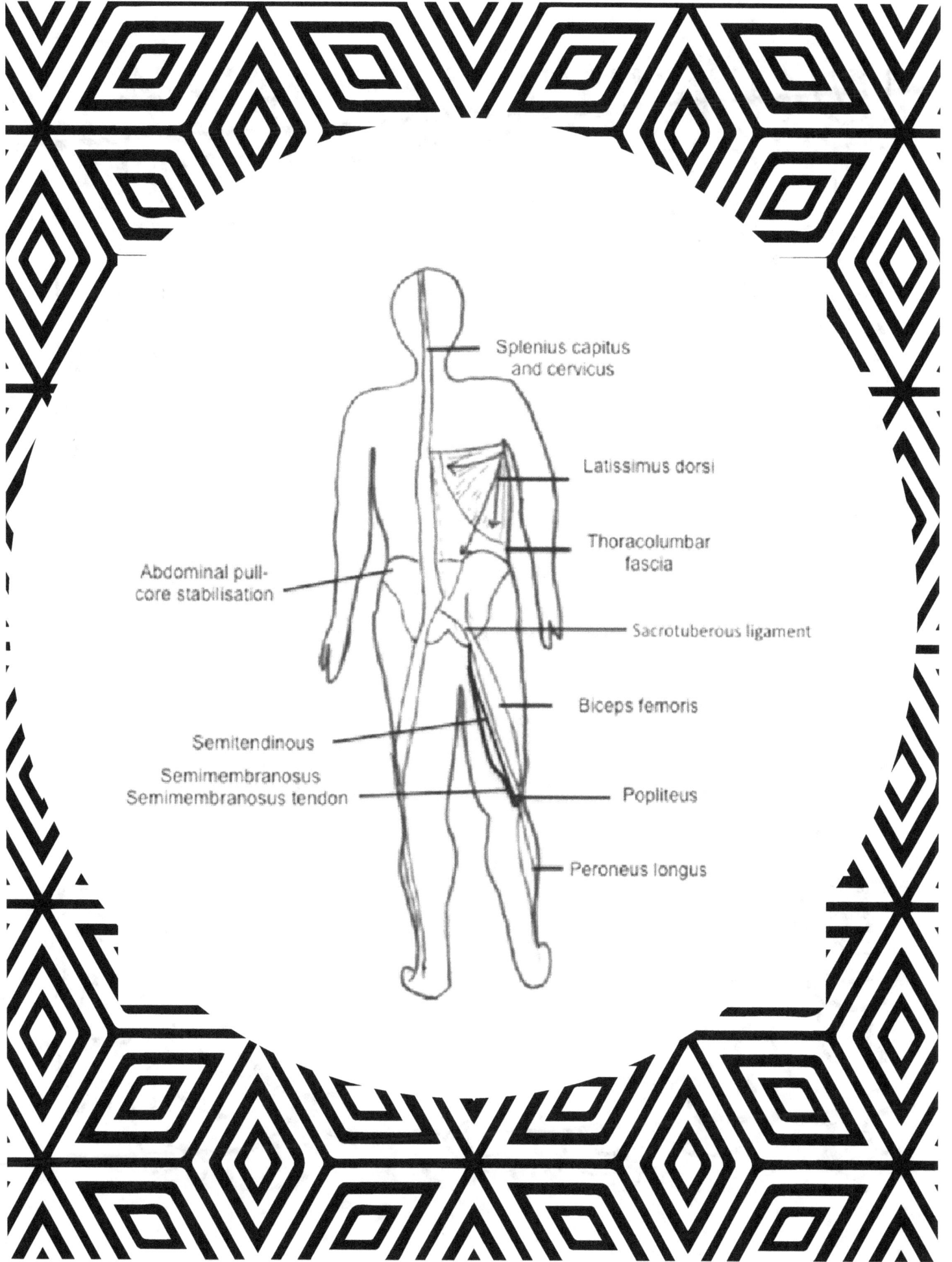

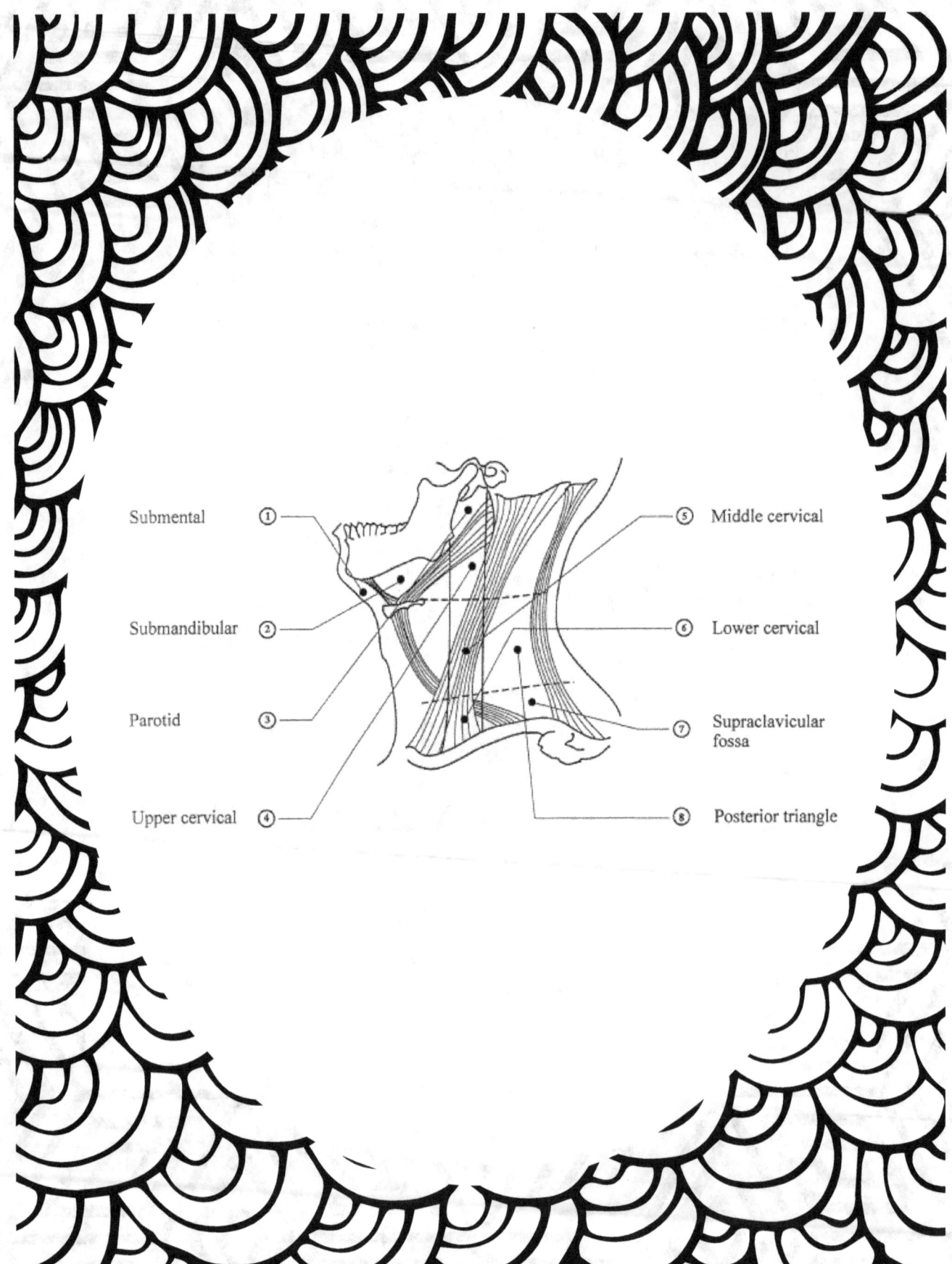

Submental	①		⑤	Middle cervical
Submandibular	②		⑥	Lower cervical
Parotid	③		⑦	Supraclavicular fossa
Upper cervical	④		⑧	Posterior triangle

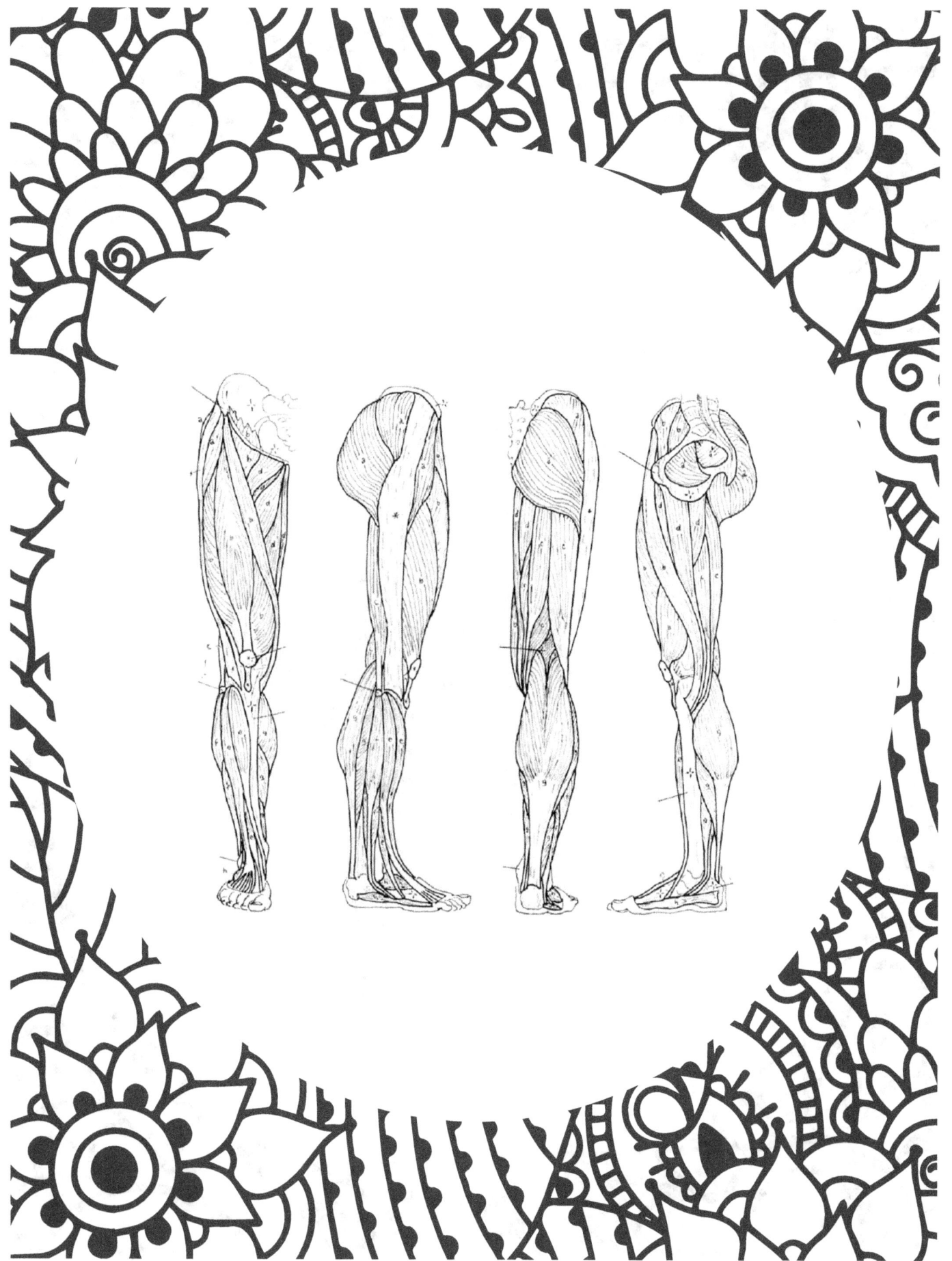

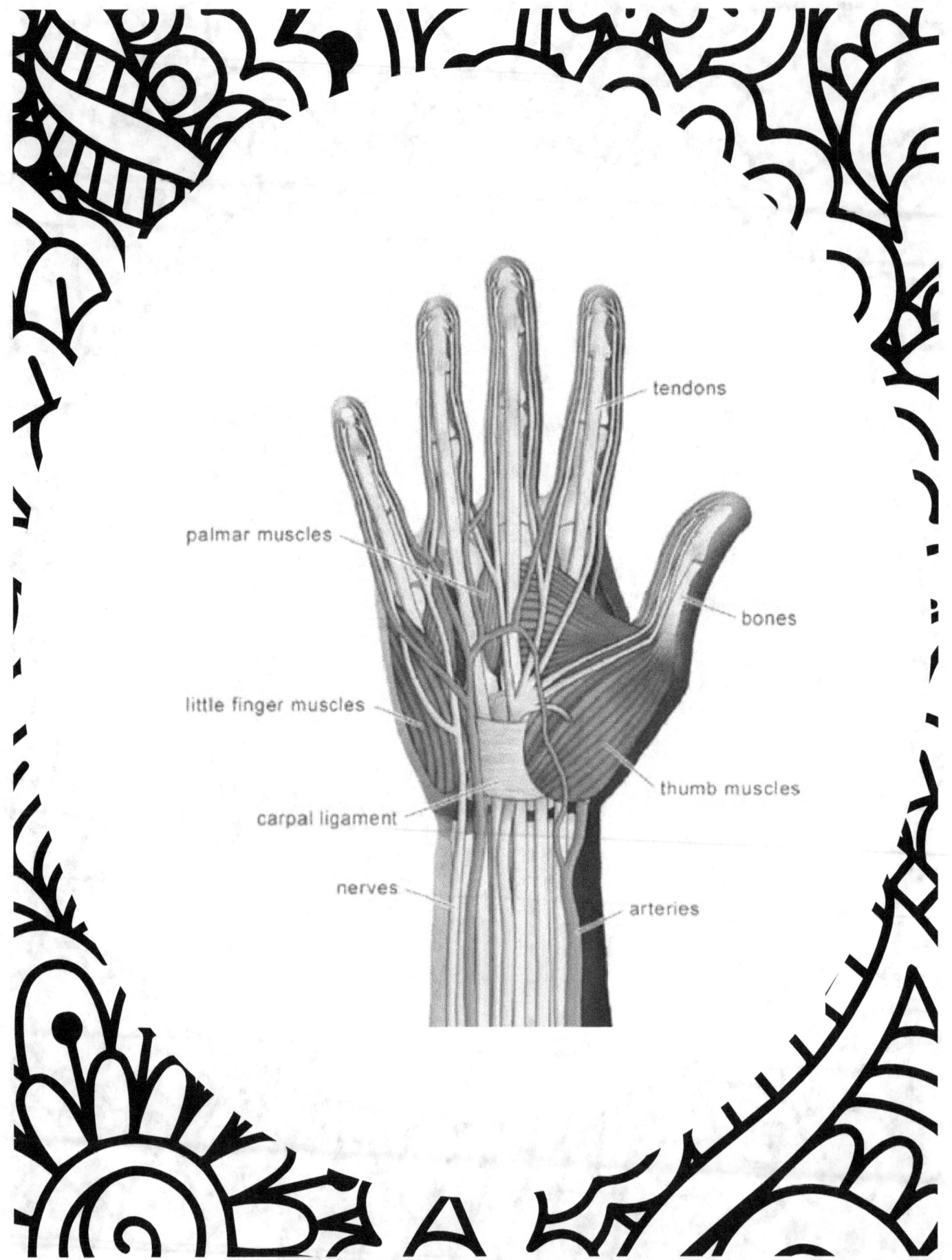

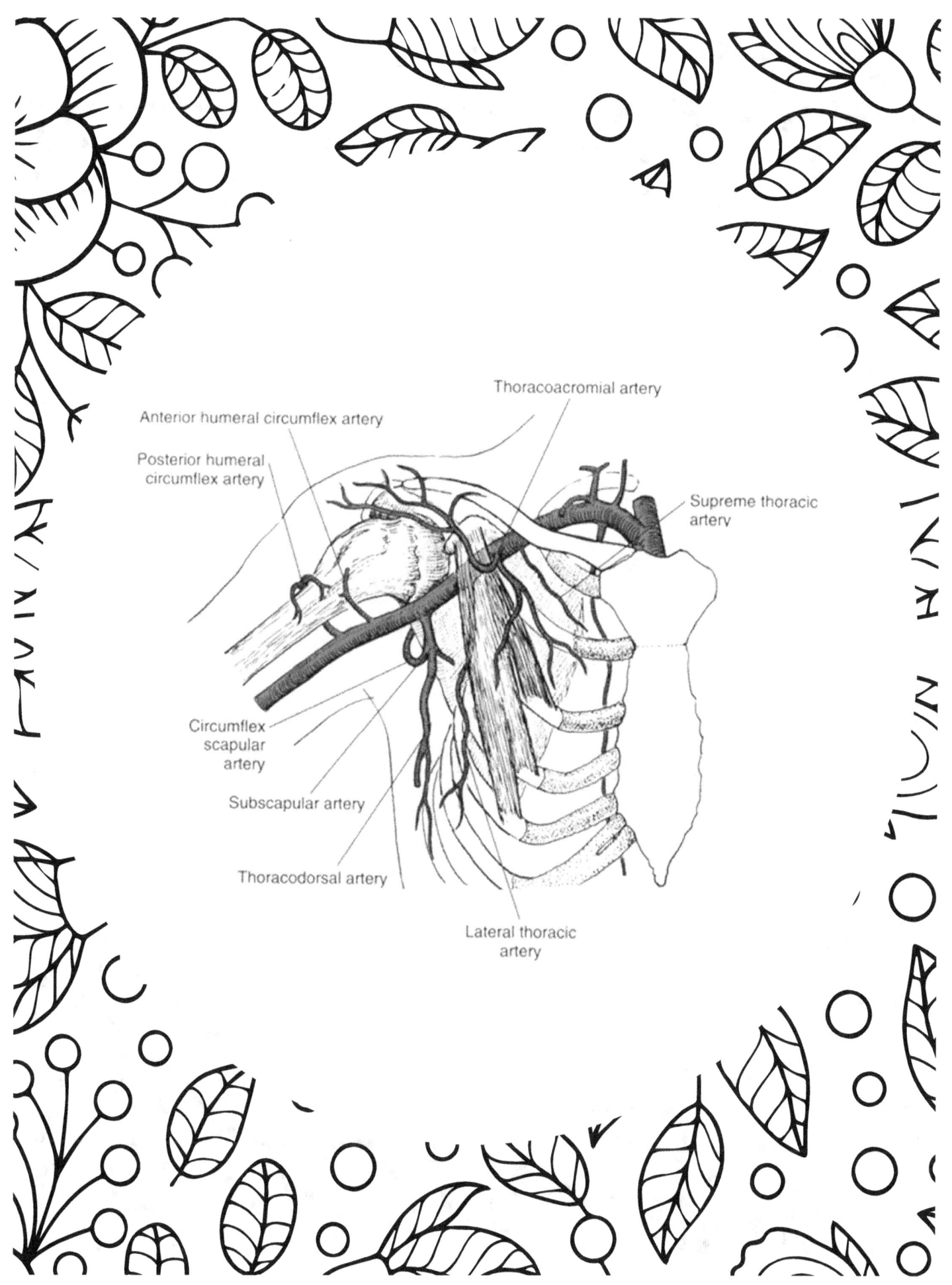

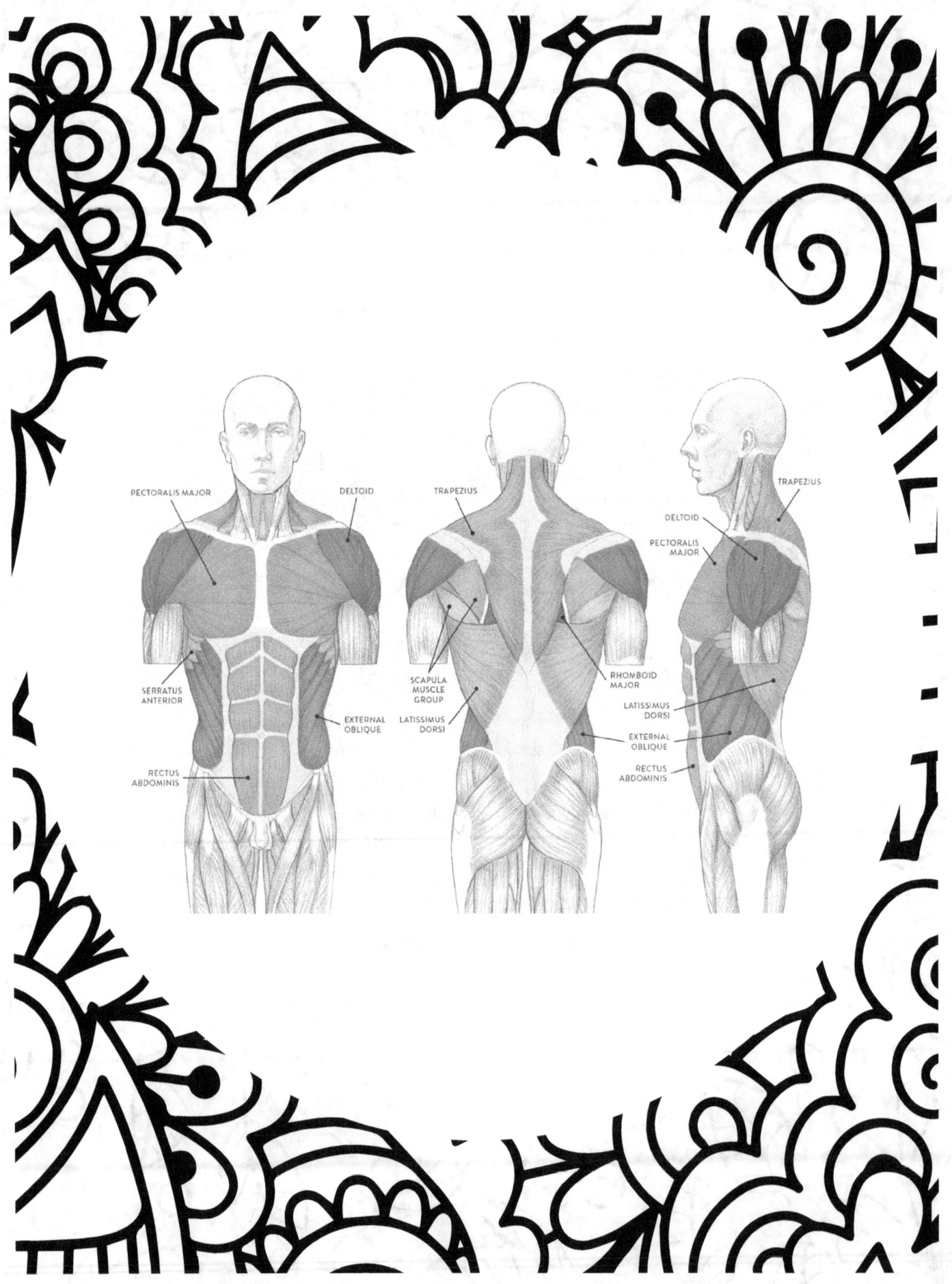

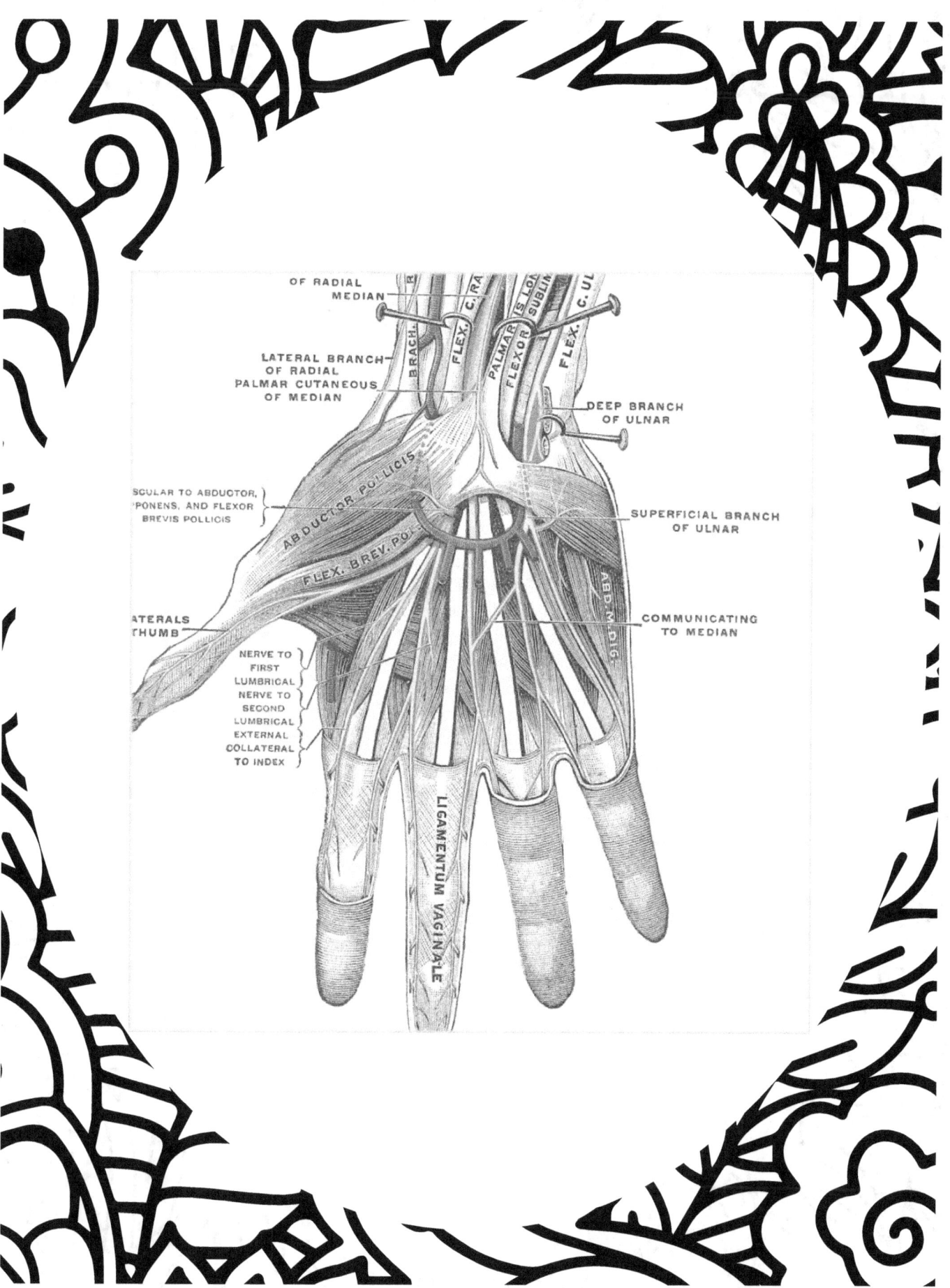

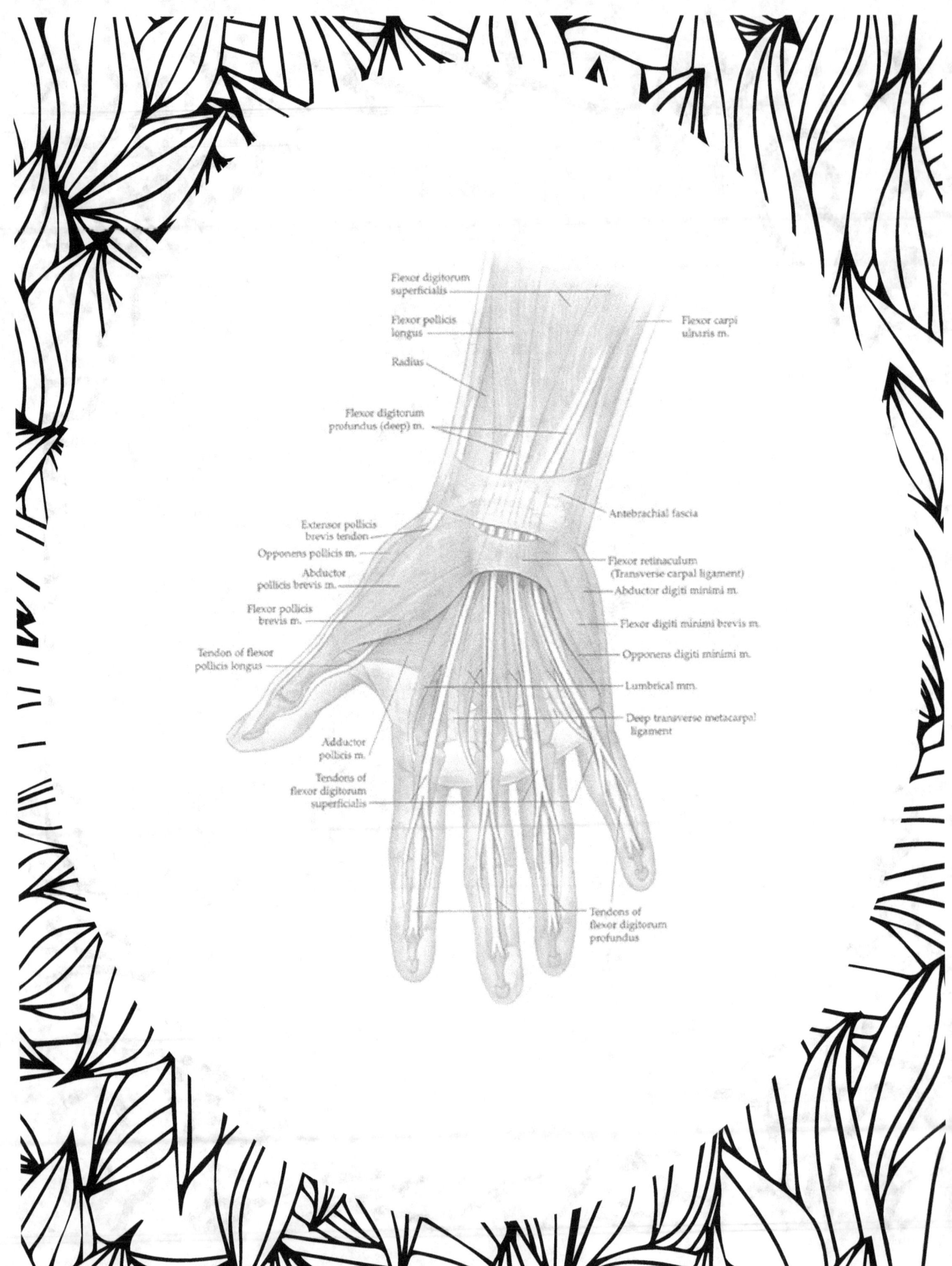

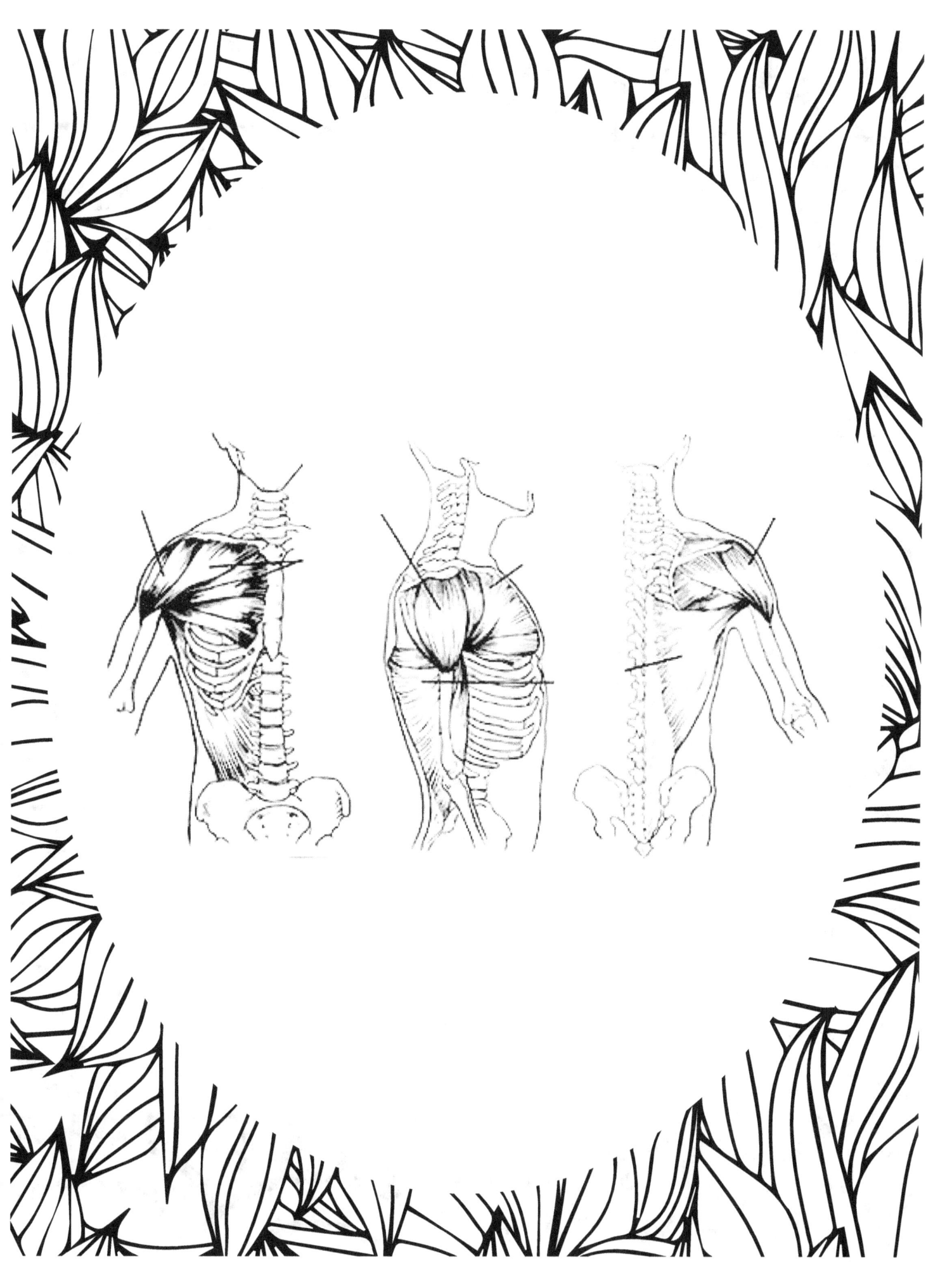

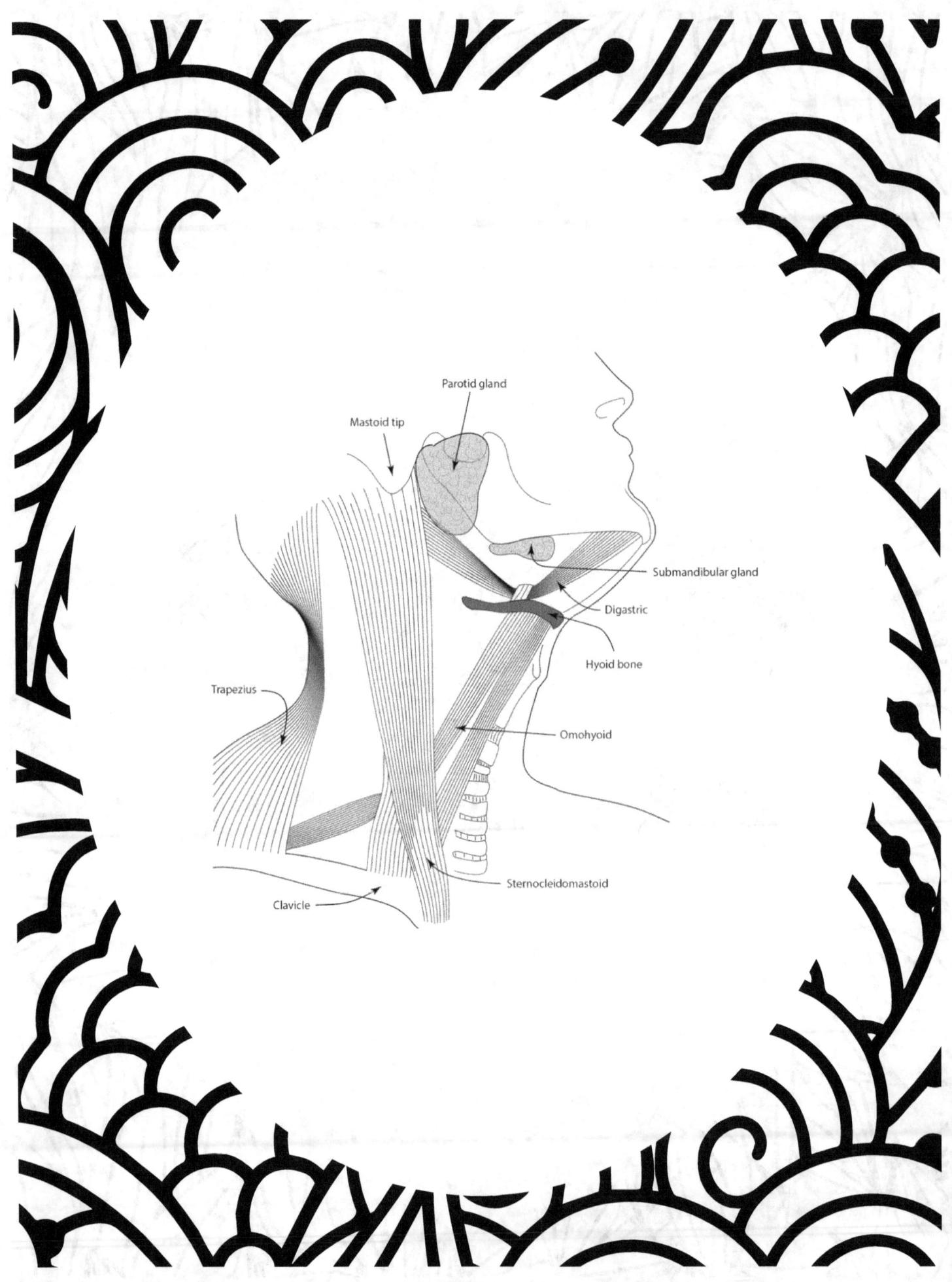

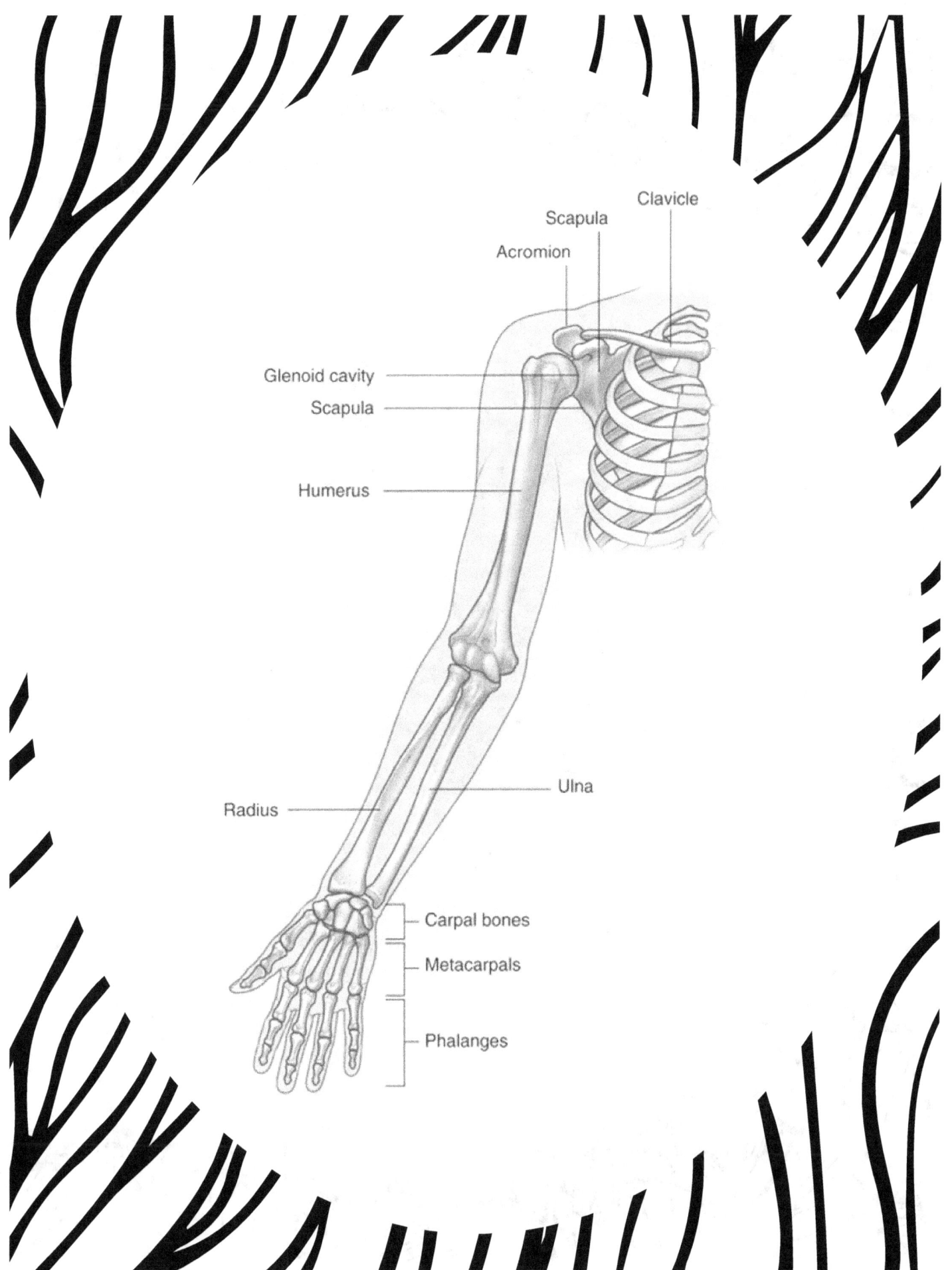

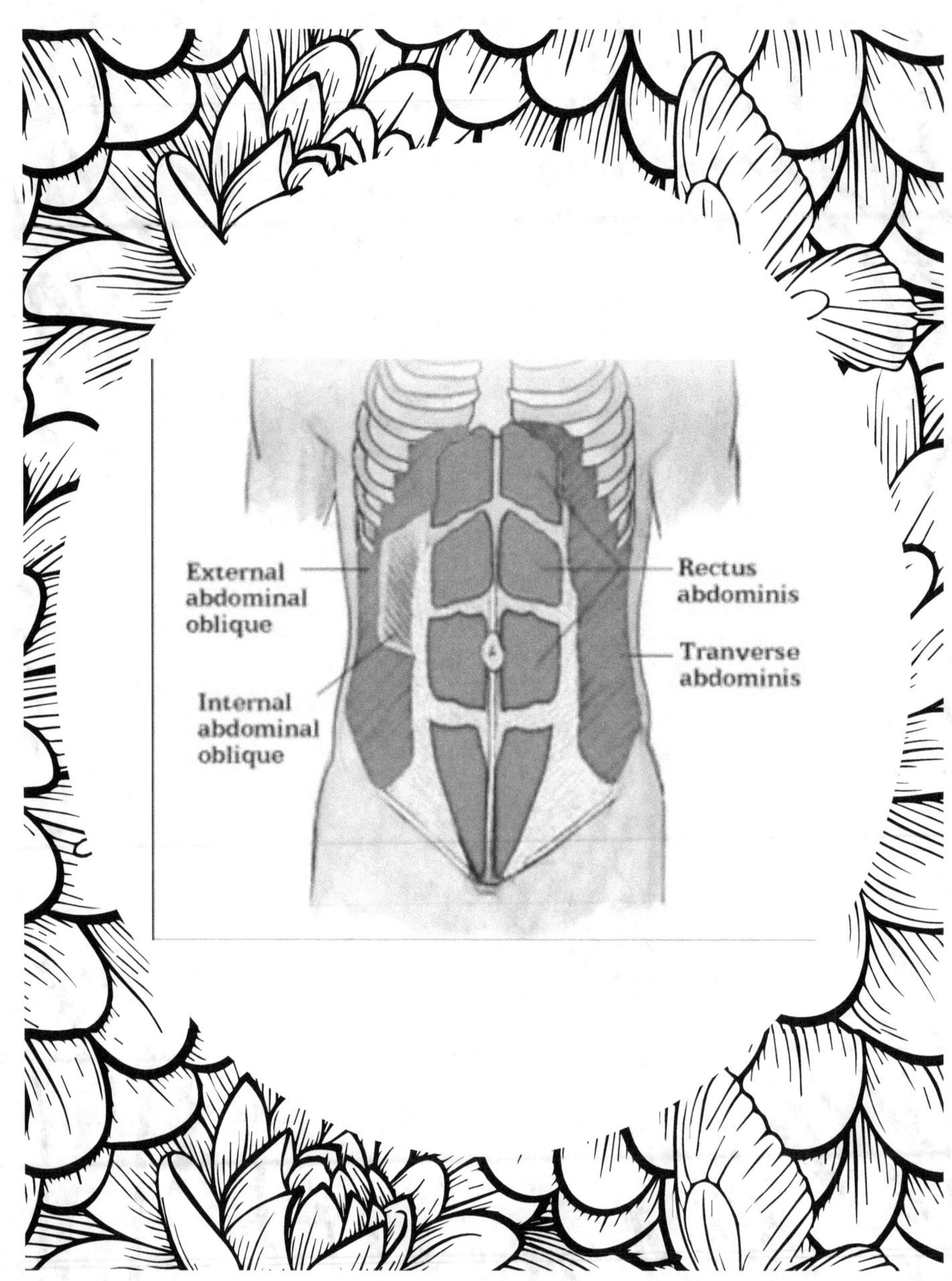

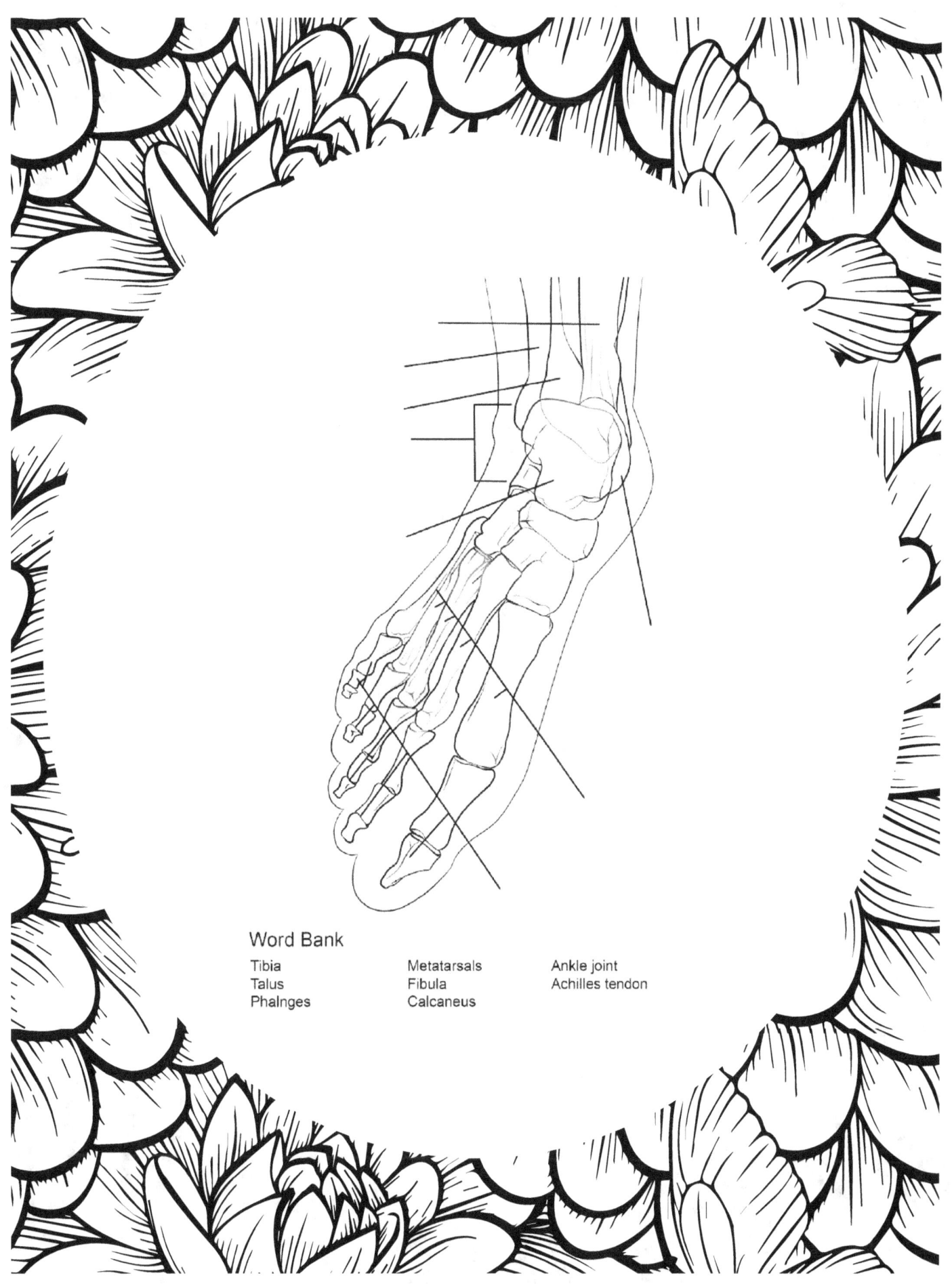

Word Bank

Tibia Metatarsals Ankle joint
Talus Fibula Achilles tendon
Phalnges Calcaneus

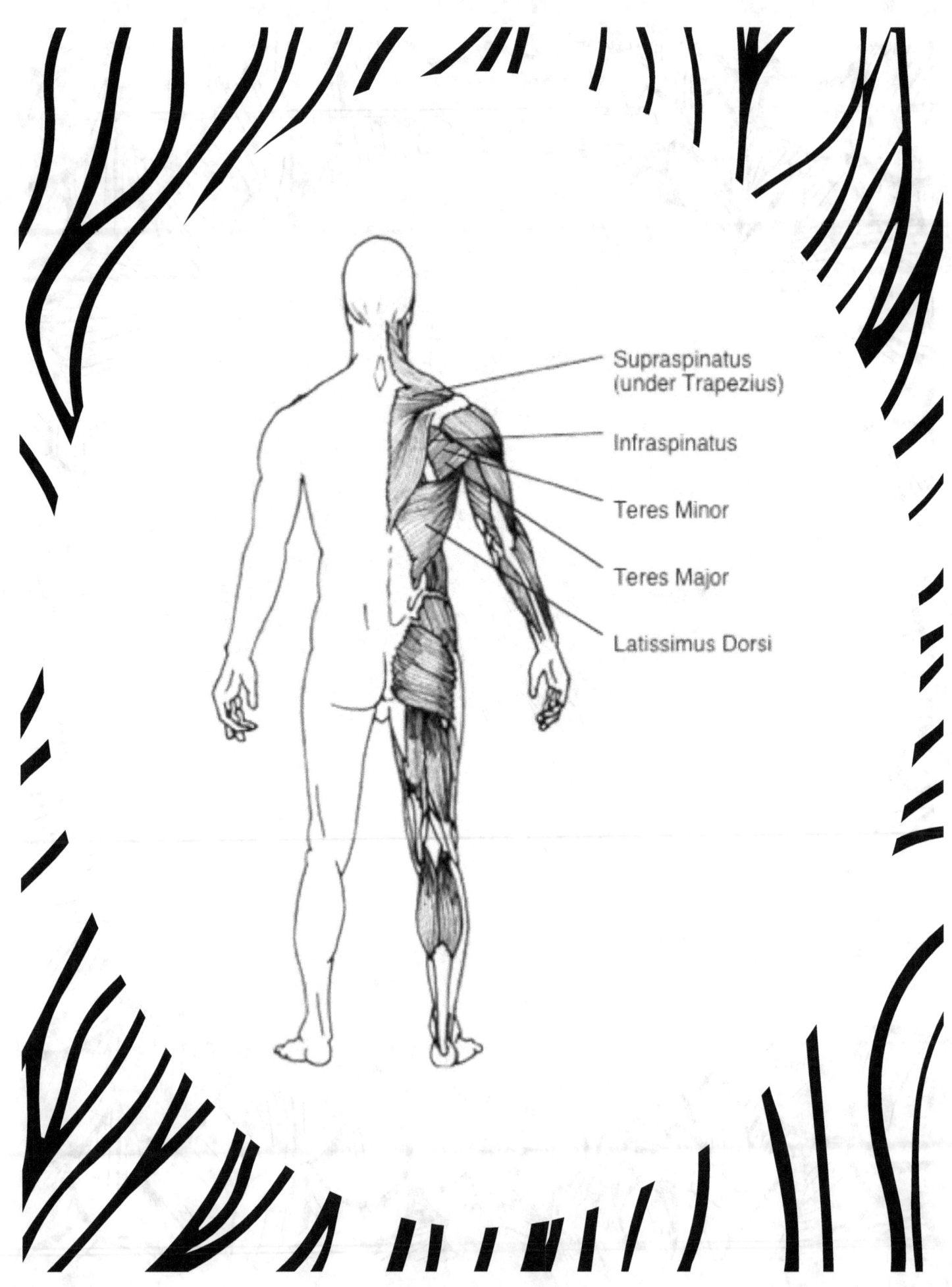

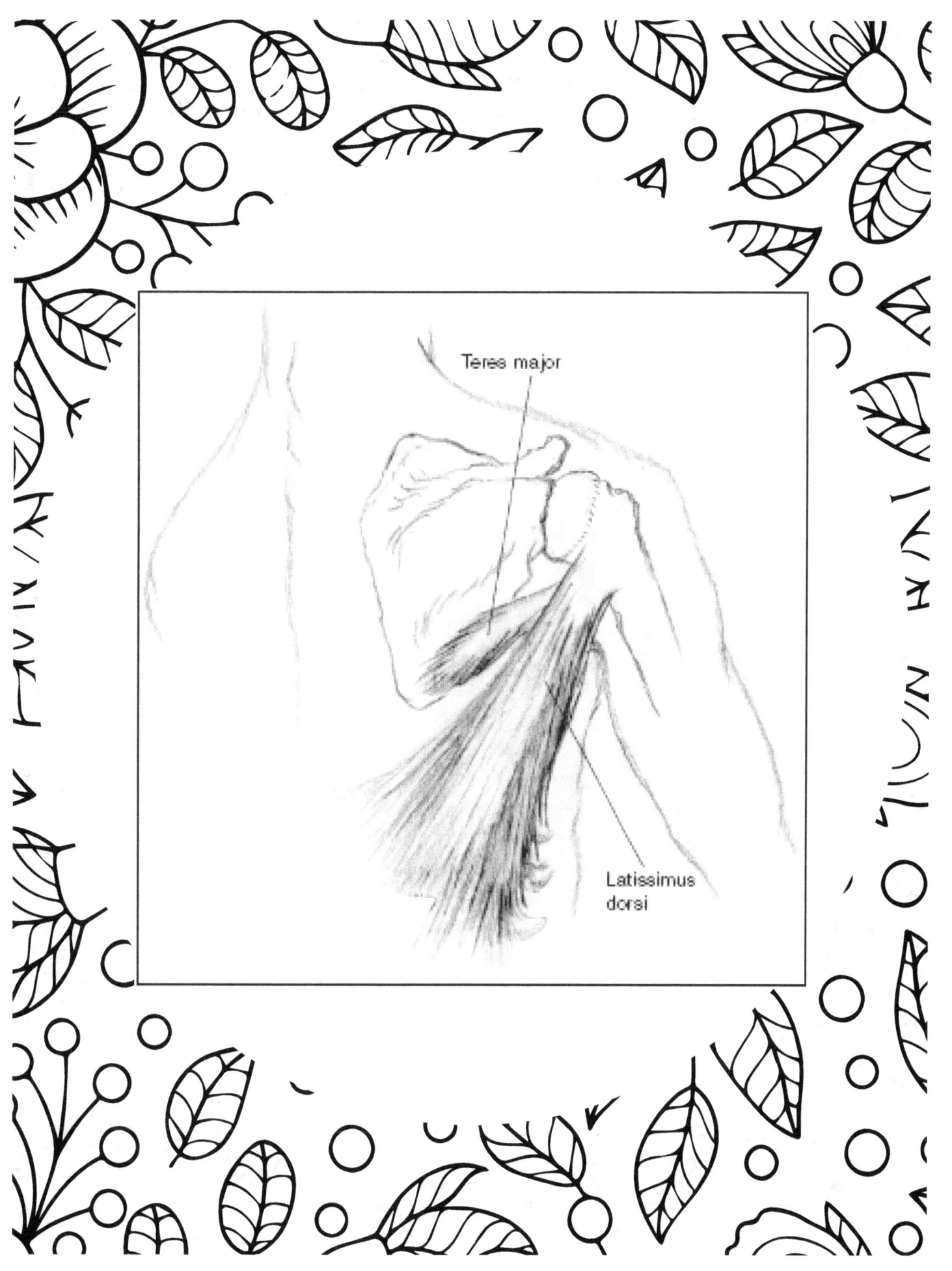

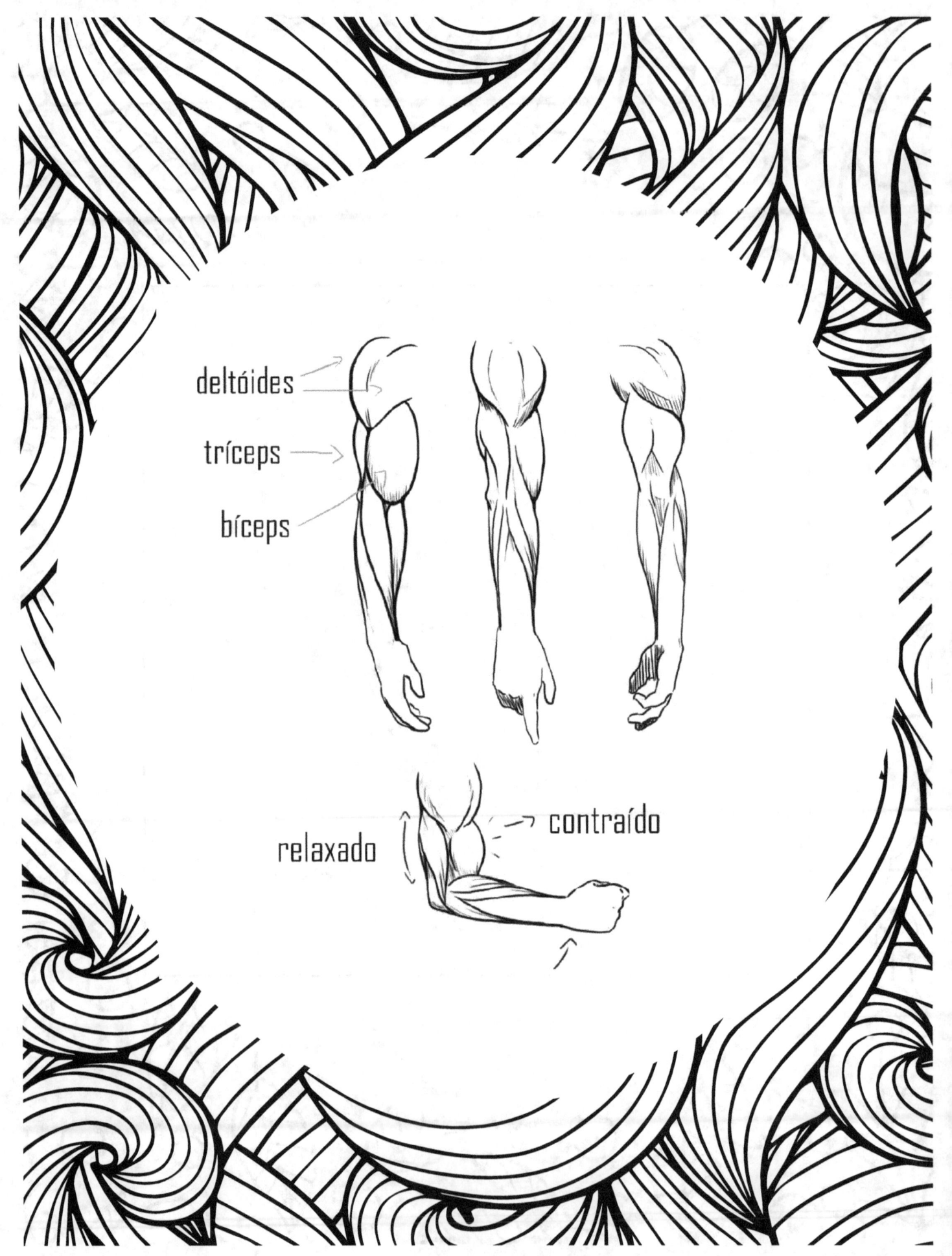

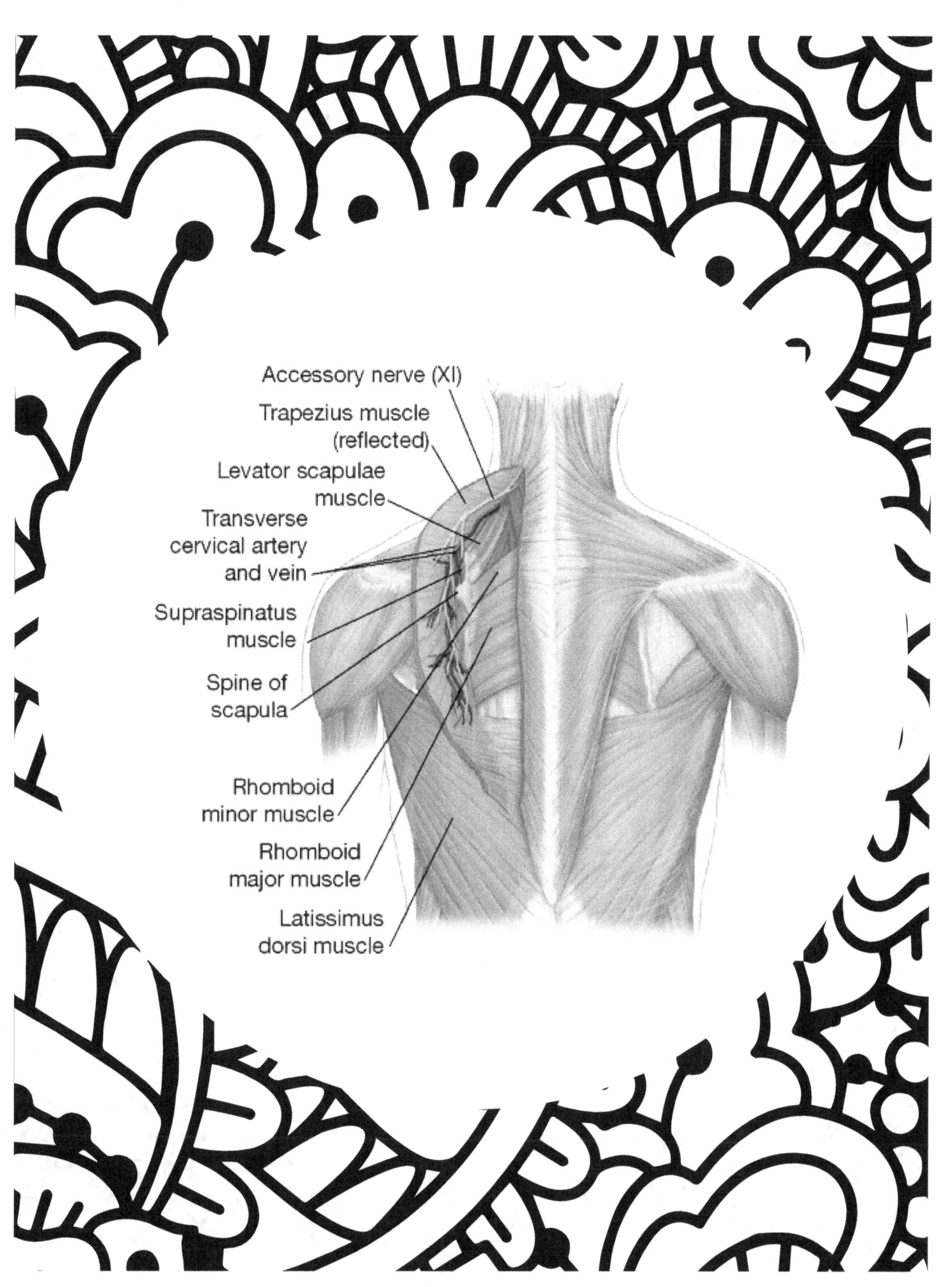

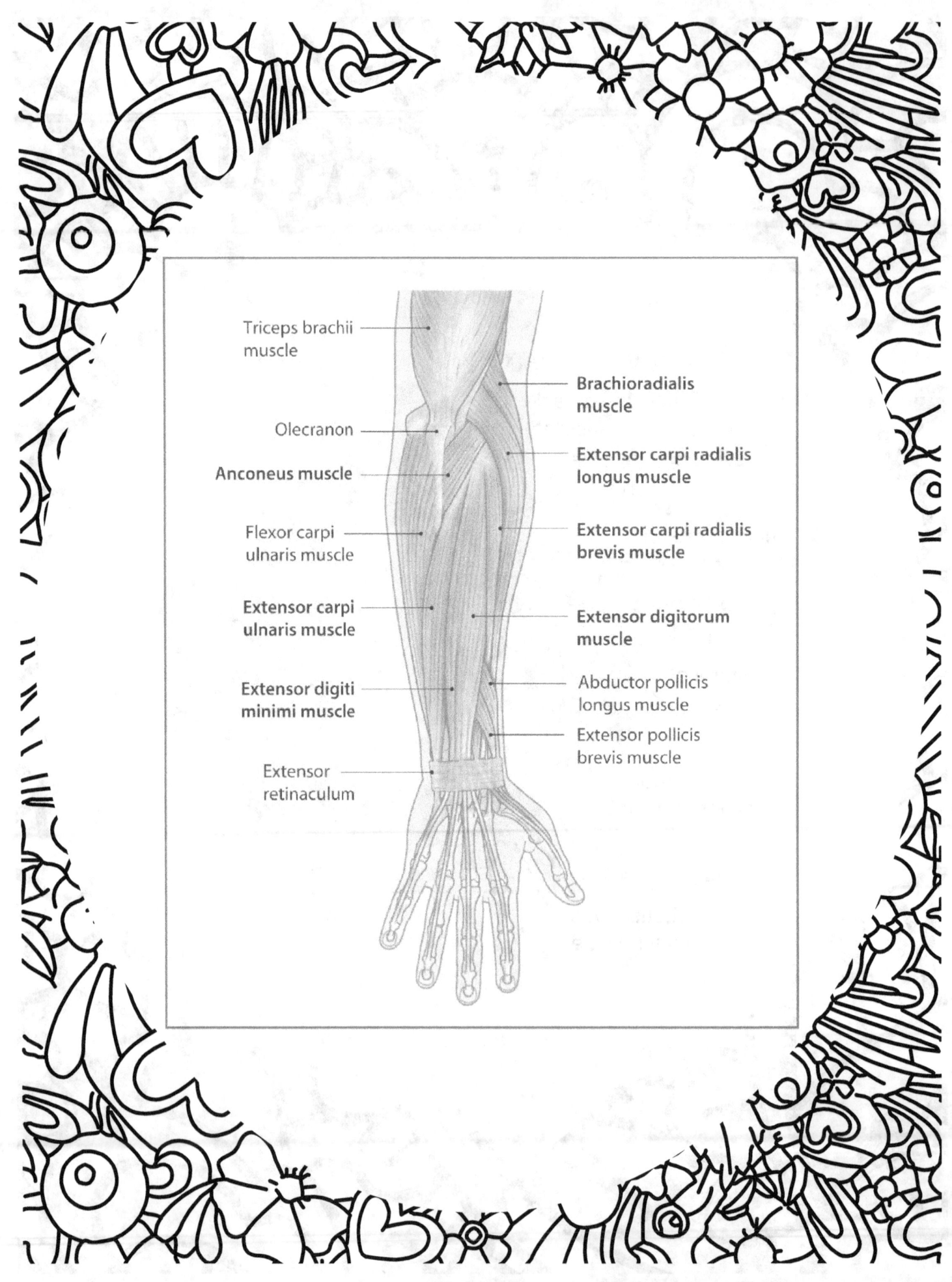

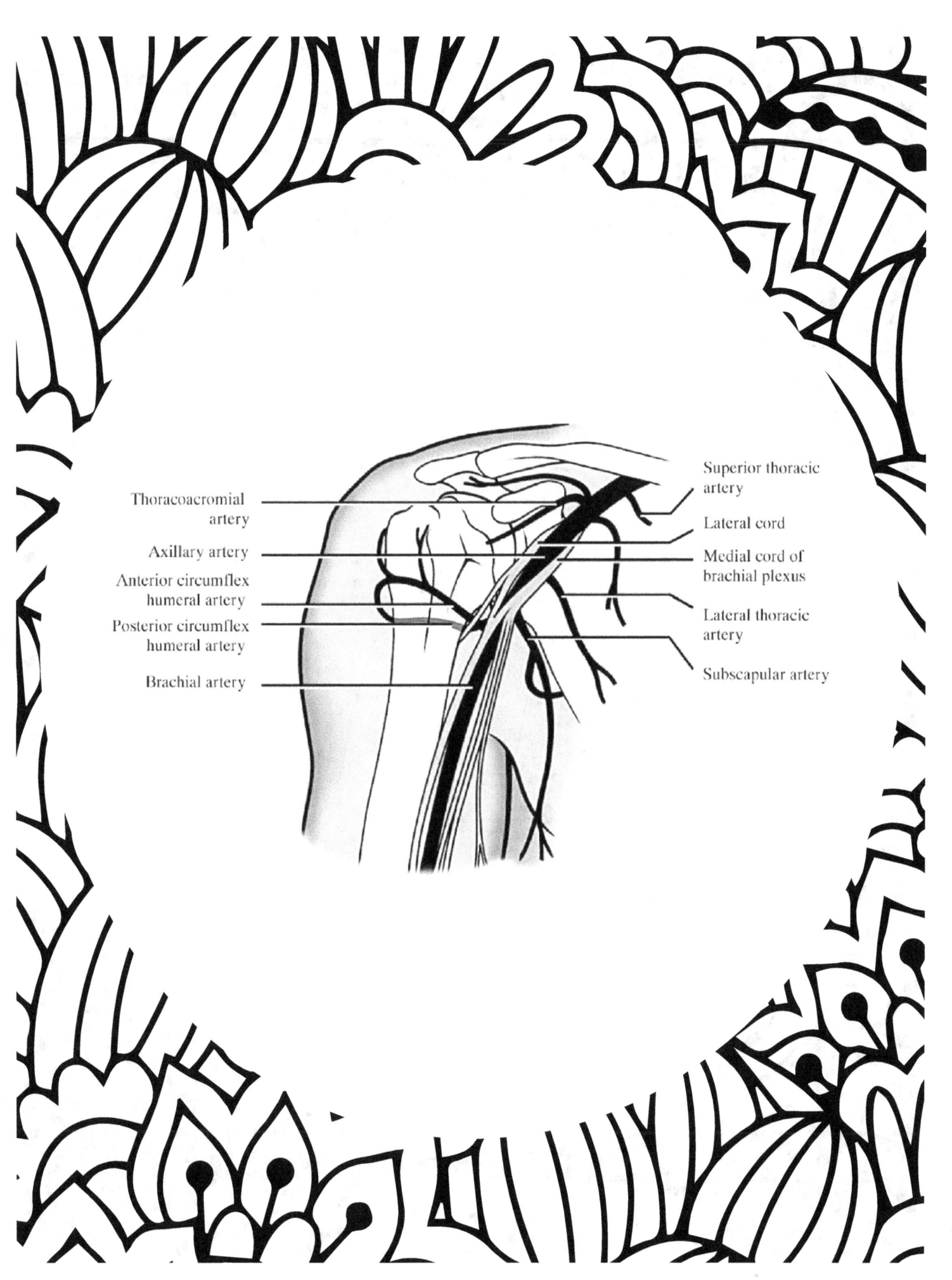

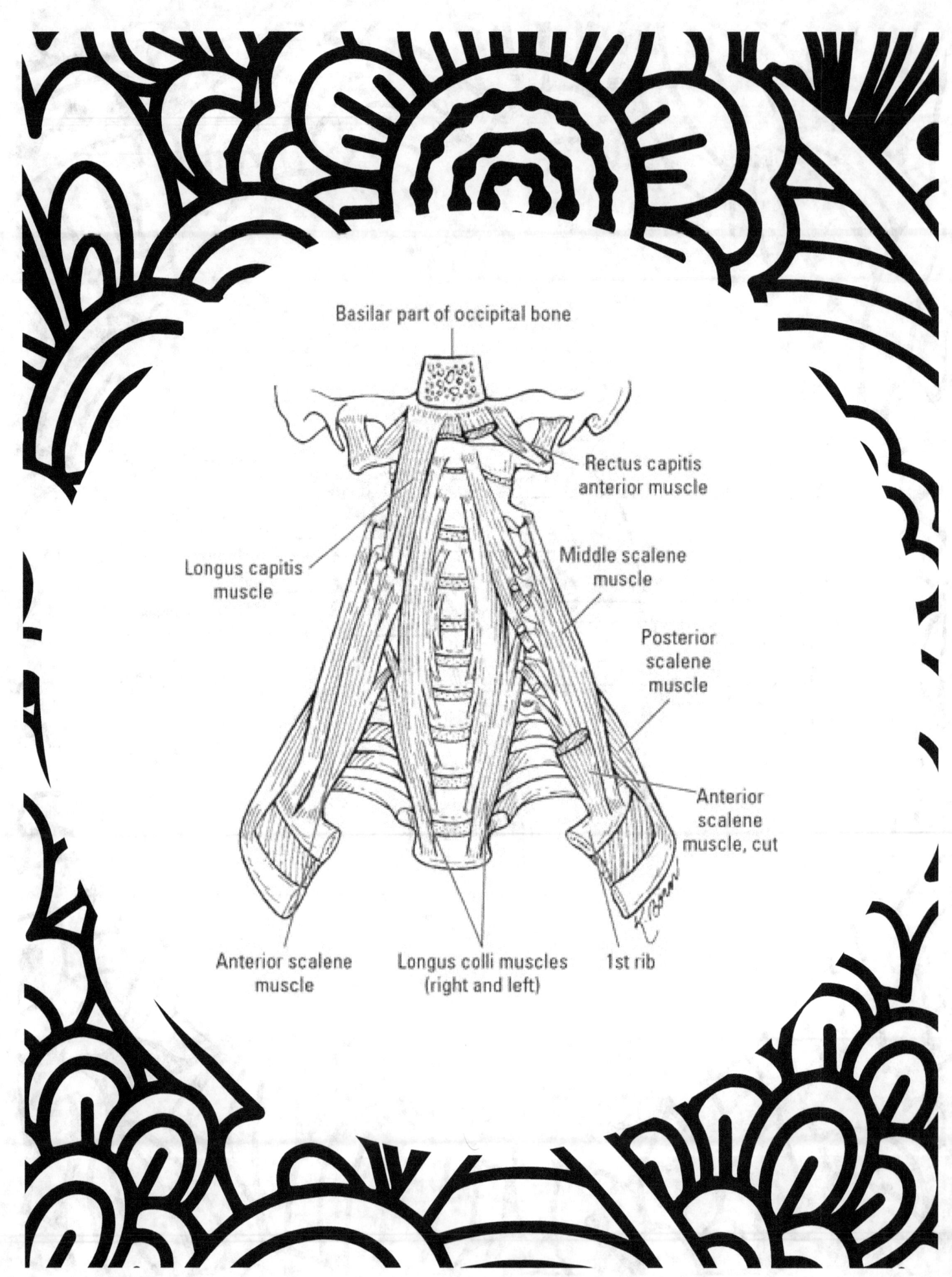

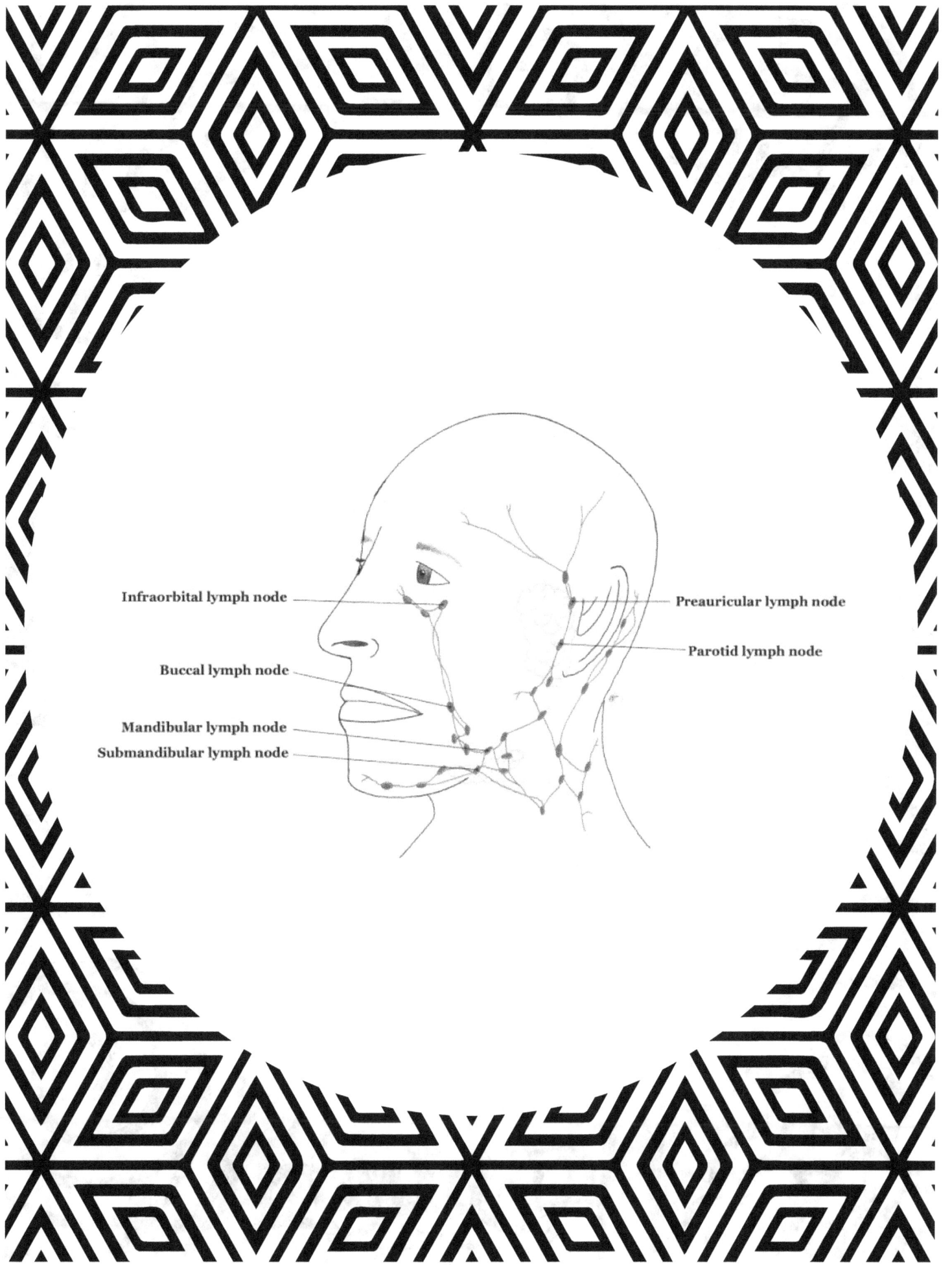

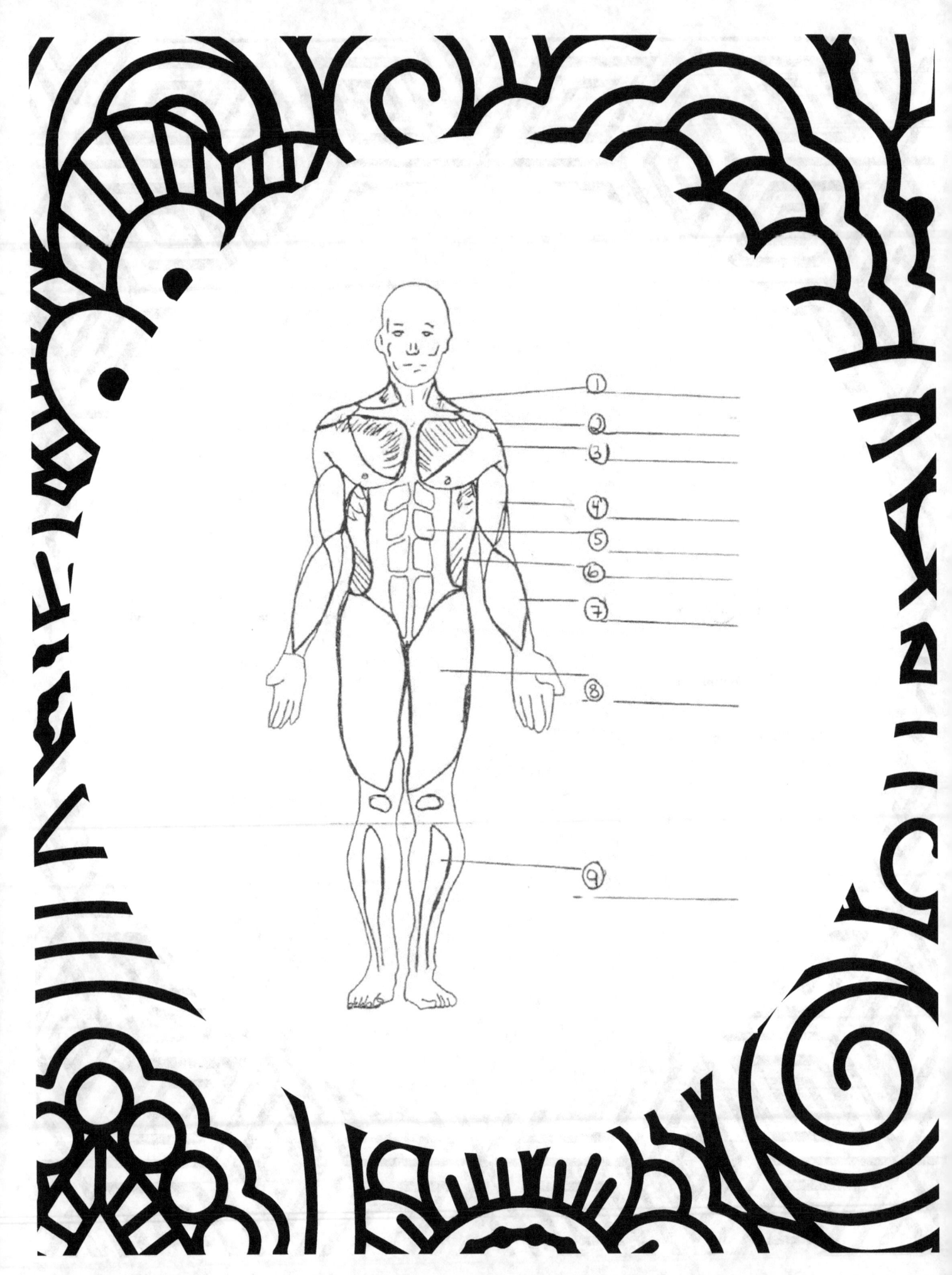

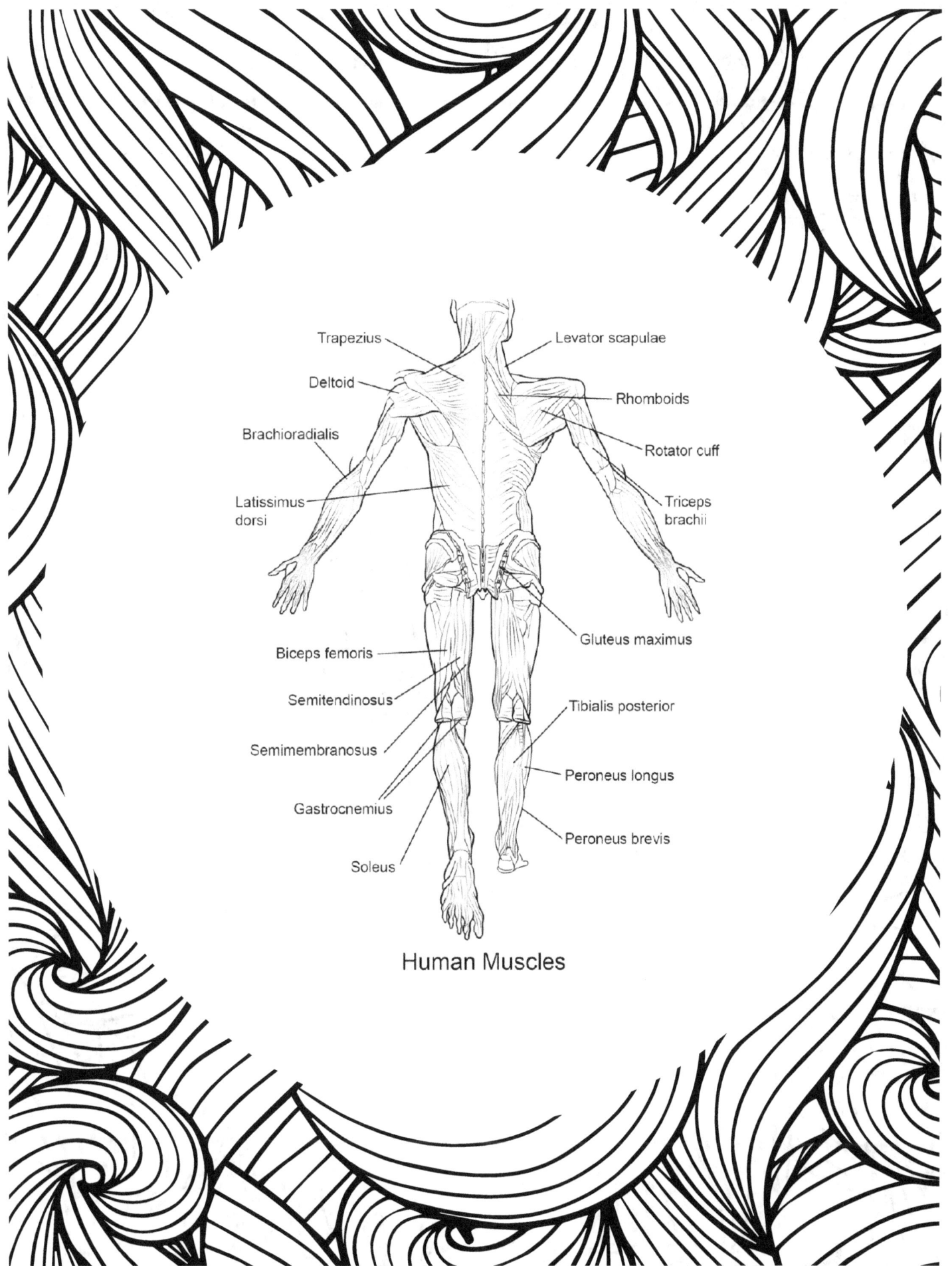

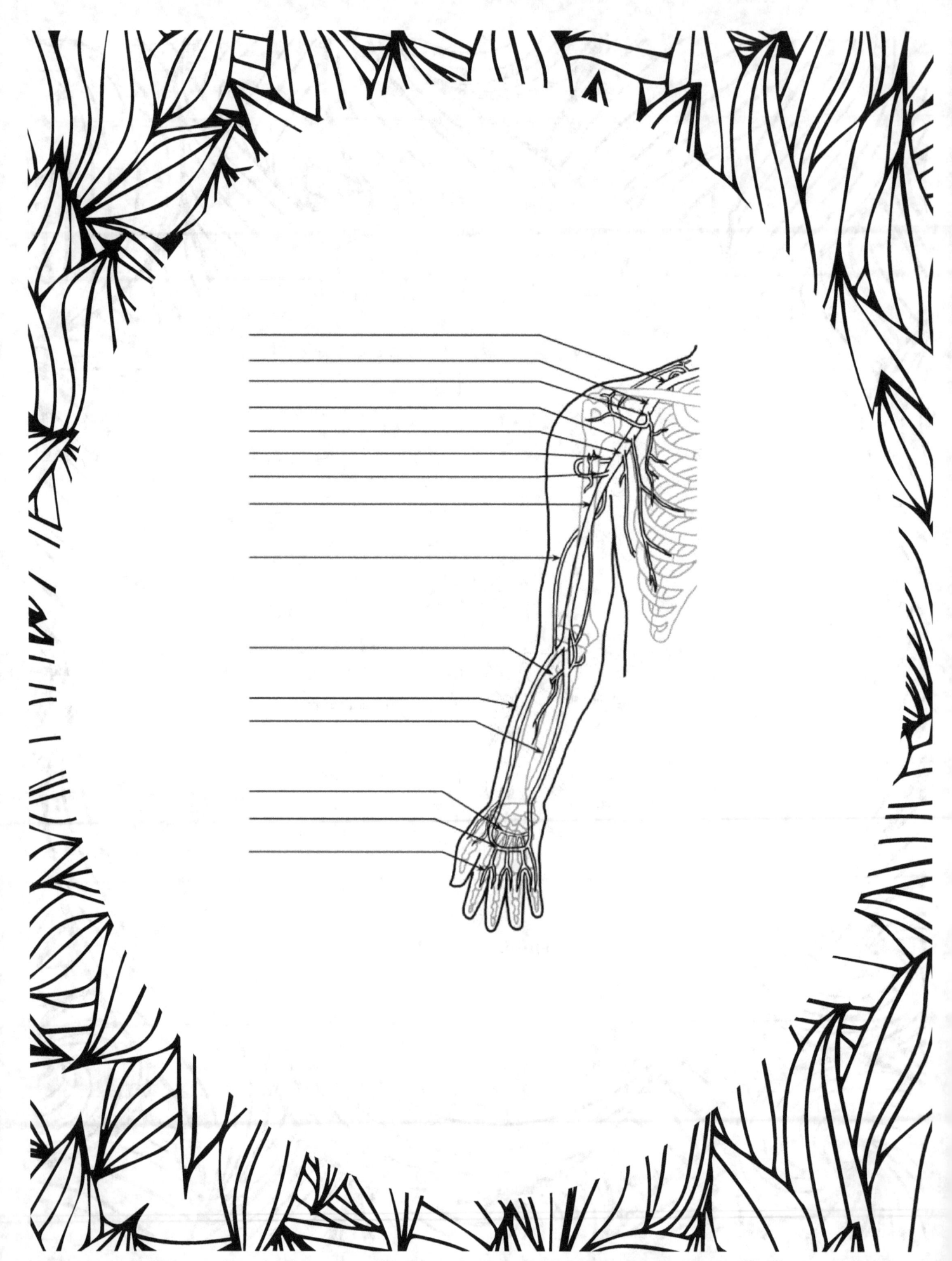

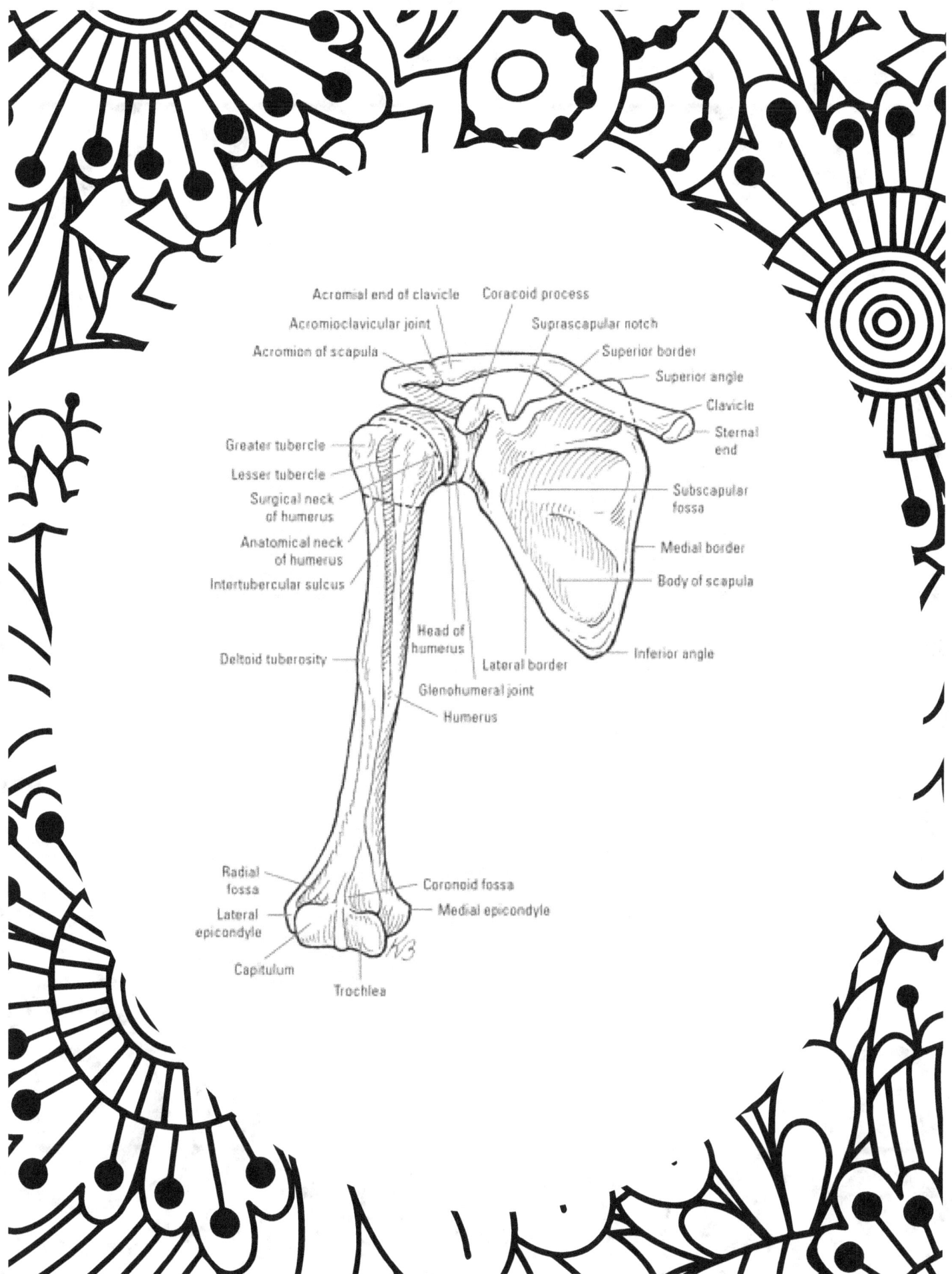

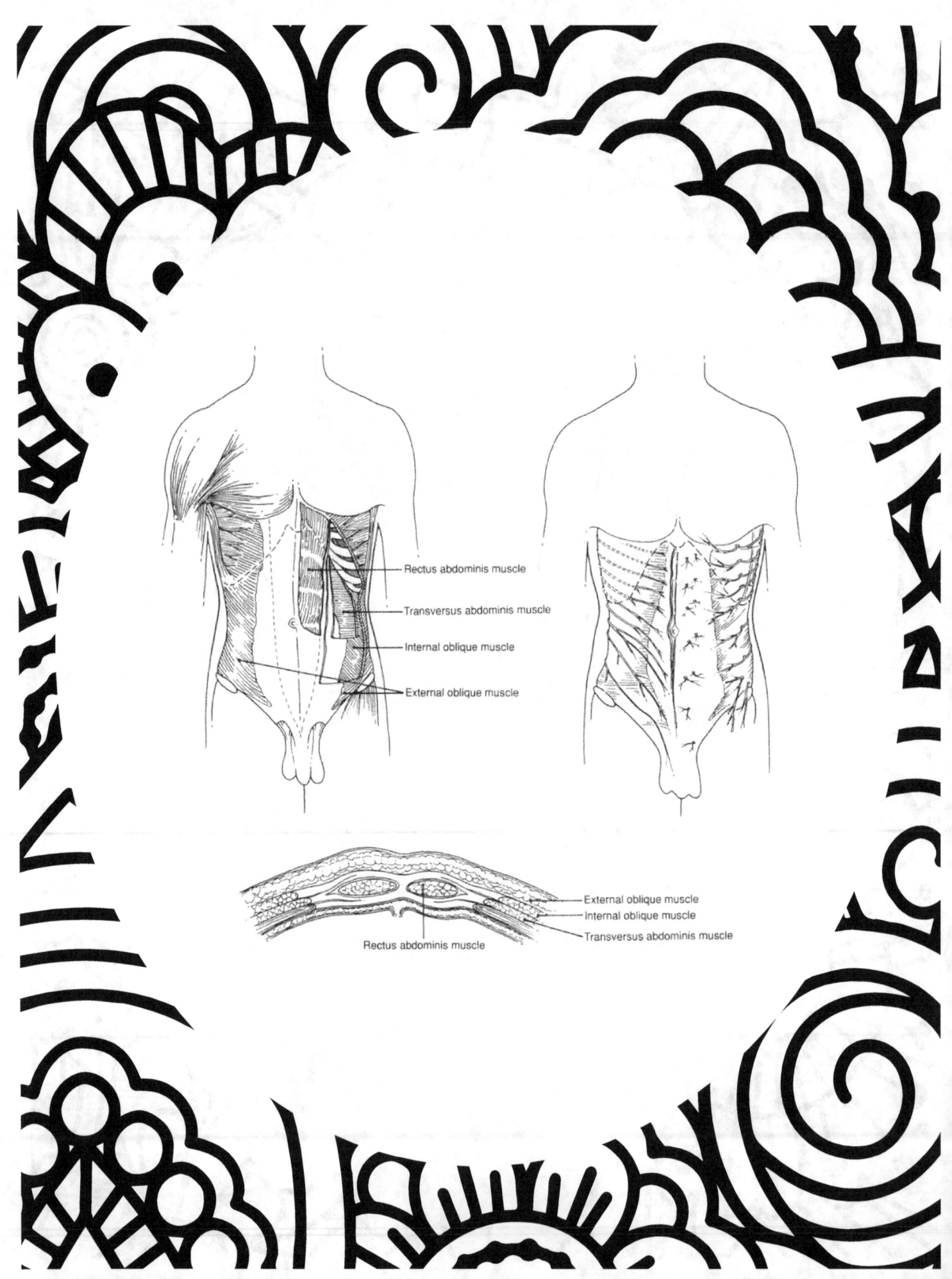

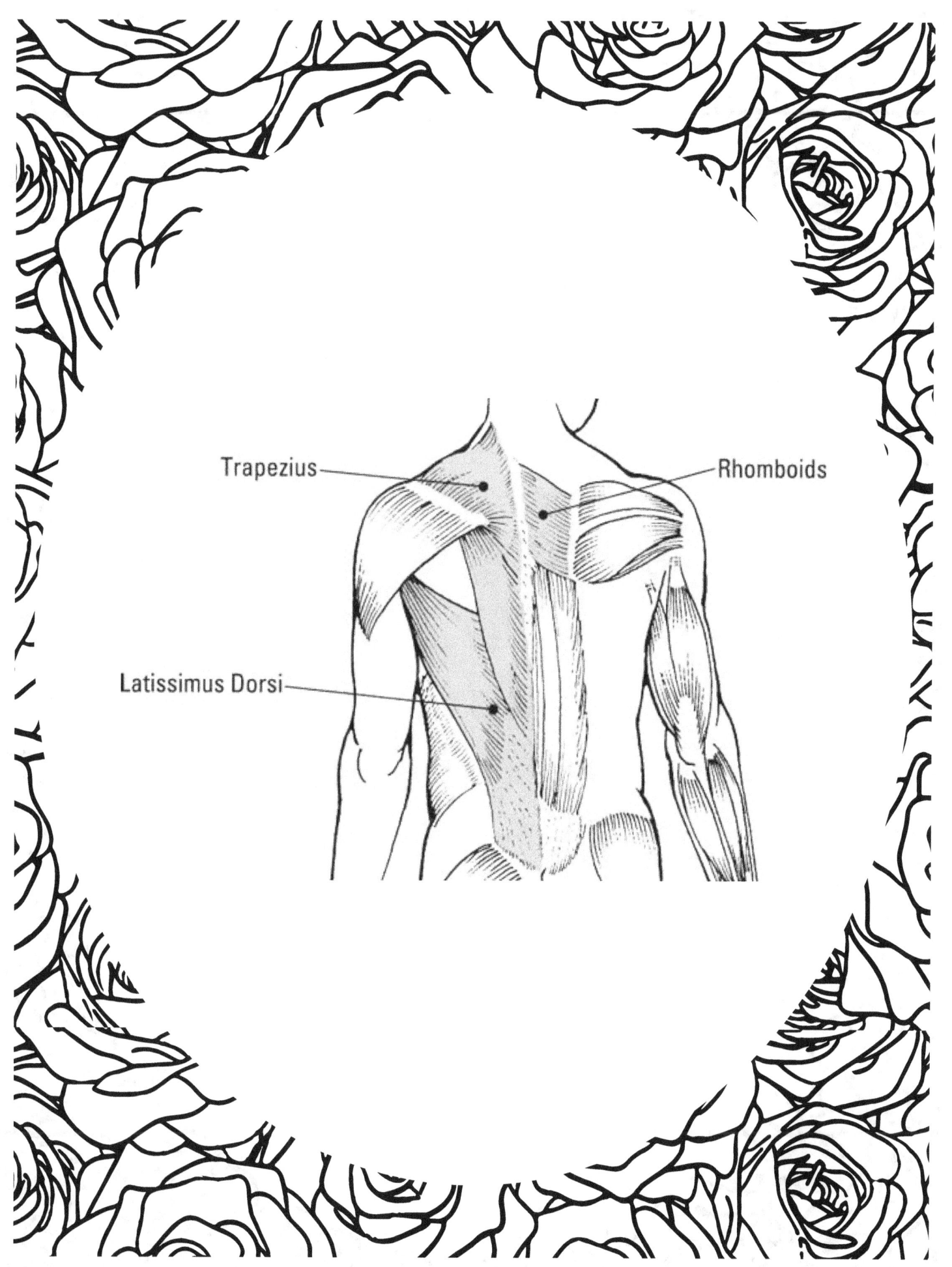

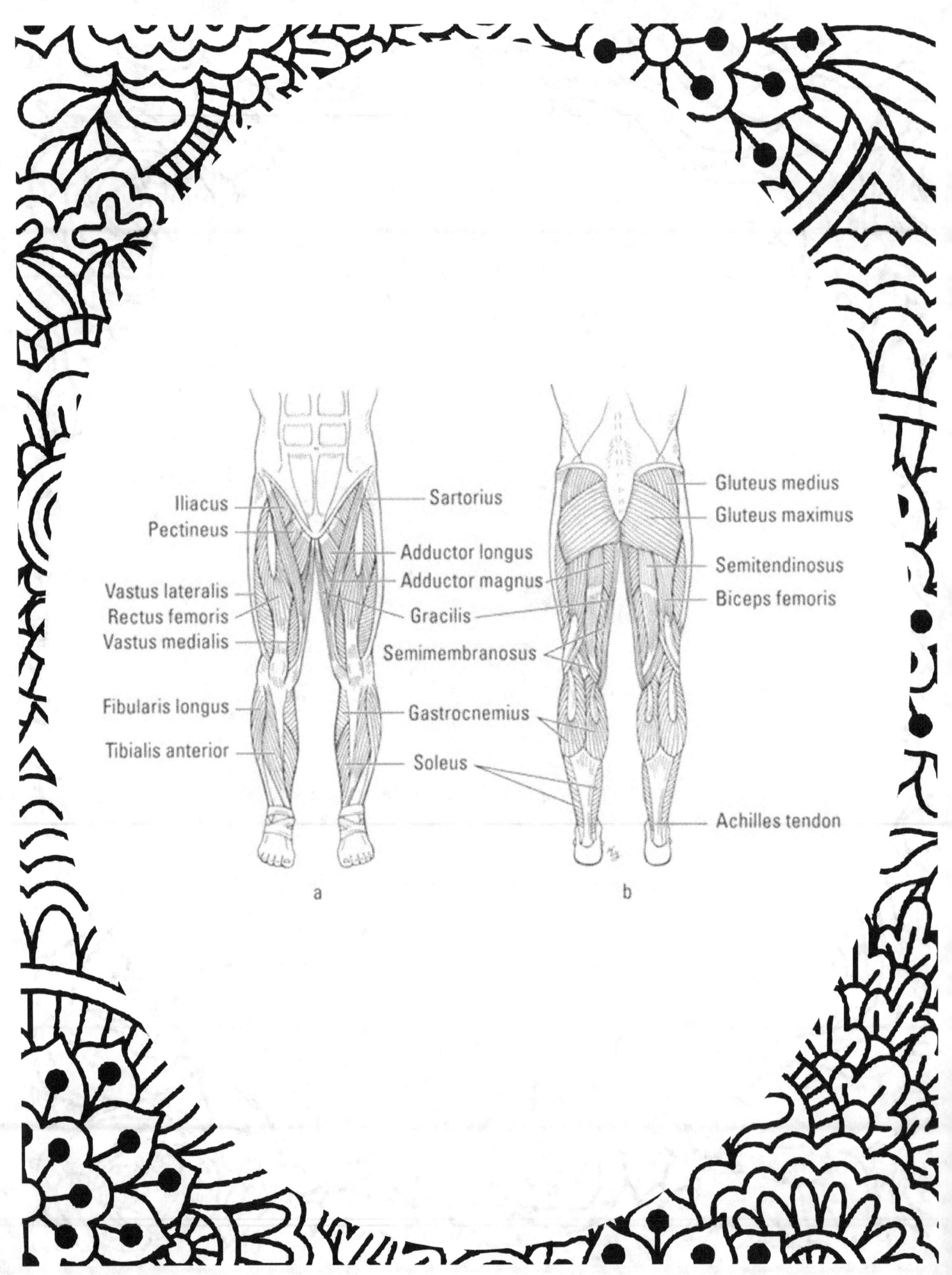